Anatomy of a Soul's Calling

Becoming the Physician Healer I Was Meant to Be

Mary Louder, DO

cairn
Publishing House

Praise for Mary Louder, DO

"*Anatomy of a Soul's Calling* reminds us that life is filled with twists and turns, but ultimately to trust that healing occurs when we align with our own timing and inner wisdom. Mary wisely relocates medicine as a relationship not only between doctor and patient but within you as a person finding a deep connection back to yourself. This book is a joy to read. Sit back, relax, and receive."

—Arielle Schwartz, PhD, psychologist, author of *The Complex PTSD Workbook*, founder of The Center of Resilience Informed Therapy

"Is there a bridge between being a physician and shaman? In this deeply personal memoir, Mary Louder gives us a first-row seat to the life events and profound experiences that led her to her soul's calling. By writing this book, Mary not only invites us to see ourselves in her stories, but also to find *our* story as we read hers. Each chapter reveals the profound connection we have with Love, Spirit, and the Universe."

—Inger D. Kenobi, author of *How Do I Look?: The Year I Stopped Shopping*

Contents

First edition

ISBN 979-8-9923836-1-4 (ebook)

ISBN 979-8-9923836-0-7 (print)

Book cover design by Mary Louder, DO

To Mom, who gave me my first push in life.

To Andy, my love and light.

To my patients, with gratitude for allowing me a first-row seat in their lives. It is an honor.

Introduction

"May you recognize in your life the presence, power, and light of your soul. May you realize that you are never alone, that your soul in its brightness and belonging connects you intimately with the rhythm of the universe. May you have respect for your own individuality and difference."
—John O'Donohue

Hello, my name is Mary. Perhaps you have heard of me.

That line is a riff on what I thought someone else once said, or at least what I had imagined them to say.

A long time ago, I attended second-grade CCD on Saturdays at our local Catholic church—those are religious Catholic doctrine classes for youth who attend secular schools. This is also known as *Catechism.* I was an eager reader yearning to learn new words and phrases. So, when the writing exercise came in the CCD workbook, the scene and question was set as follows: Jesus and his disciples were in a boat on the Sea of Galilee. When Jesus came ashore, a crowd had gathered. They were eager to hear from Jesus and his disciples. The workbook prompted, *What do you think Jesus said to them?* My reply was written in my best penmanship:

"Hello, my name is Jesus, perhaps you have heard of me."

I think my mom spit out her coffee when I read my homework aloud to her. You see, I loved using the word *perhaps.* That was the entire origin of my reply: word usage. It was completely lost on me that Jesus was the Son of God and all. I thought he would just use the word *perhaps.* And I did not quote any ancient text, as I don't think the word *perhaps* is even in the King James translation. Perhaps.

That phrase I wrote in my workbook has remained a mainstay in my vernacular throughout my entire life. It really seemed to tickle my mom's funny bone, as she frequently reminded me of the story all throughout her life.

And, really, that is what my book is about: the story of my life. A memoir. Brené Brown says that maybe people's stories are just data with a soul. We connect with stories because they are about people, and stories are rich with emotional data. In that case, I have a lot of data and stories and soul all wrapped up and ready to share.

Perhaps, had I written this book much earlier, you would have only a short story to read, with a few data points. But then I would have left out some of the good parts. I seem to have lived a lot of life in my short time. My hope is that you not only see yourself in the stories, but also that you find *your story* as you read mine. For me, that would be a success, a connection with a deep and abiding revealing of our souls, together as humans. Together, through our stories, we understand and connect with ourselves and with others. Connection is in our wiring.

Writing a memoir is cathartic; it is healing. However, before the healing, it can be challenging. Facing many of life's events, decisions, ups/downs, and, well, just life can be quite daunting. I decided to write with reckless abandon and face the regrets that I have, the doubts that I lived and perhaps (see, there is that word again) may even still possess. What I learned for sure—and now have what I call *a felt sense of*—is that no matter what turns, decisions, detours, success, near-death experiences I have experienced, I always was connected to Spirit. Love was a constant, holding me, the Universe, and all of its infinite wisdom and presence. Love was with me all of the time. I was never separate from Love/God/Spirit/Source, whatever we may call it. I was never separate. At times, it felt as if I was. However, upon reflection, I was not. It was only my perception. It was not true, *not my truth*.

That was not what I was taught in Catechism, or later in my life, especially as a Holy Roller or an Incredible Woman of God (IWOG), or even one who eventually seemingly threw the baby and the bathwater out. I was never separate. I was never lost. I was never in need of saving. That simply was not true. I have heard it said that a miracle can be described as *a change in perception from fear to love*. That seems right. When I was able to see that the many fears I held onto with a firm (read white-knuckle) grip were what often kept me from that connection with Spirit, and then from connection on the inside with the three Ss: spirit, soul, and soma (body); when I found that sense of connection on the inside—mind, body, spirit—I was not afraid. It was a miracle, I was at peace, and my body responded with a much more regulated neuroendocrine immune system. (More on that when we get to the medical bits.) But suffice to say, I was hitting on all cylinders and cooking with gas!

As a physician, I live by the creed that if you listen to

the patient, they will tell you what is wrong with them. That is an idea from Sir William Osler, one of the fathers of modern medicine. I believe when you hear a person's story, you are hearing data points, you are hearing the emotions and connecting the data points, and you are seeing who they are as a soul, a spirit, and a body. What a joy and honor and privilege that is. It never gets old. In writing about my life, I listened to my stories by writing them down. I saw areas in which I needed healing, by reconnecting various aspects of my heart and soul, wanting the war within to quiet so I could find peace. The answer was not outside of me (an external locus of control) but rather within me, in the interior of my soul, spirit, and soma (body). By harmonizing those pieces and allowing connection to Spirit, I found my way back, and my body has healed and is continuing to heal. So, in a way, this memoir is about self-healing. Not to be confused with self-help, but self-healing. You could say this book is about "physician, heal thyself" and how, in doing so, I found keys and steps and ways to deepen my practice as a physician and more tools to help patients heal as well.

The body has the inherent capacity to heal. That is how it was designed. We don't sit around and stare at the cut on our finger, hoping it will heal. No, when an injury or cut occurs, we provide first aid and then set the stage for the body to do the healing. We don't even need to have it in our consciousness. We may, in the form of concern or even worry, but that can slow the healing process, interestingly. Sometimes a willful neglect is the best approach, and the body inherently heals. In the same manner, sometimes letting life itself sort itself out is the same thing. I have found that to be true. After certain traumatic events, it was all I could do to put one foot in front of the other and then, somewhere down the road, I found answers. Or, sometimes, when a live event happened, I needed support then and there. And then life sorted out.

Making meaning of life is a different story, however. This is where you actively reflect, observe, and, hopefully, understand your life and its twists and turns that provide the meaning. I believe everything happens for a reason and that life is meant to be lived in a transformative fashion. We have, or at least can find, lessons in everything. In every day that we live, we can learn, grow, and change. That's not to say that there's anything wrong with us if we don't see a lesson, but we can grow in understanding, insight, awareness, and perhaps even enlightenment from everything and everyone. Trees, plants, rocks, animals, and people are the others we interact with, and their circumstances and our encounters with them all bring messages to us, if we listen and if we are open. That is the connection I long for, first with myself and then with all the others.

What I learned in writing my story is that each chapter of my life has an arc, an entire storyline, and then an epilogue. Then the epilogues seemed to have a similar thread, and that is where I saw that I was never alone, I was never away from love/Love or spirit/Spirit. What got a bit confusing was understanding my connection to self and the soul, and certainly to the body part of self. At times, I found myself at war with my body; at other times, bewildered by or with my body. And sometimes, dissociated from my body. To me, this describes the human condition. I believe our goal is to live in harmony with ourselves and everything that surrounds and envelopes us—all of nature, and all of humans and their nature(s) as well. We are all connected, rooted, genetically more alike as humans than different, yet our expressions of these genes are as wide and as varied as the number of people that there are.

As my life and, therefore, this story and memoir unfolds, I trust that you will be encouraged, entertained, empowered, and, hopefully, enlightened as to the power of your own story and presence in the world. It is a unique time to be on this planet and that thought is not lost on me. We have a lot to do and to be responsible for, while—at the same time—we are meant to live fulfilling and enjoyable lives. I believe we are meant to live abundantly in our relationships, in our businesses, communities, and circles of influence. It is no use trying to be anyone else except the best version of yourself, because, if you aren't you, nobody else can be you.

It took some time for me to come home to myself and my "Self." However, in each instance, when I did return to me, my life was fuller, richer, and more connected. I have come to realize that once you are connected to yourself, not only is it the safest place to be, but also the best place to be, because from there, you can go anywhere.

So, grab a cuppa your favorite brew—mine is an Americano with a splash of cream—and sit a spell. Read and enjoy, as this data with a soul is dedicated to you from me.

With love,
Mary

Prologue

Eight Minutes to Spare

It has been a minute since I started this book, while I took a minute. I took a hiatus, but now I have returned to finish writing. You wouldn't know this unless I told you, so I am telling you: The vast majority of this book was written and then I chose to stop writing for a season. They say that sometimes life gets in the way of your plans. Well, that certainly happened. What started as an adjustment to my supplement products and sales of the supplements took my business and vision in a whole new direction. I wasn't afraid to finish this book or to "put my story out there." No, I just made a choice, a business choice to add an online store to my business. No small task.

Opening a virtual online business (again) took months of planning, executing, tweaking, and more tweaking... and did I mention the tweaking? The project required all my creativity and energy, and I chose to put my book on the back burner. Notice that I used the phrase, "I chose," because that is true. It's not as if things just got out of hand, or I got distracted from the book. No, there were multiple points where I consciously decided to hold off on writing so I could focus on business-building. Gradually, as the business adjustments, growth, and associated projects were accomplished, it became clear that the missing piece was my story, my book. So I returned to complete that which I had begun only a few months before.

On the day I returned to the book, I determined that I would write all morning and into the afternoon, starting early. I wanted zero interruptions. Sounds like a great plan. The actual day started with me briskly hitting the snooze button and rolling over for an additional hour of sleep, snuggled in with my husband Andy. It was dark and dreary out, and I felt no need to rush. Then, after getting up, I made an eggnog latte and I tackled the inbox, just in case.

That resulted in both some rabbit holes and some very good things being accomplished. But the morning was ticking by.

I had felt that, before doing any of that day's writing, I also needed to take time to complete a shamanic journey so I could reconnect with my guides—those helpful others and beasties who have accompanied me on this journey. Earlier in the year, when taking a memoir writing class, I learned how spirit animals are guides for any aspect of our lives. We did a shamanic journey to see if we met up with our own *beastie*, a spirit animal guide for our book. The journey resulted in me becoming acquainted with a beastie that felt in alignment with my writing. What seemed to show up for me was a female tortoise. Her name is Lucy. I see her as an old, wise tortoise, with a great big shell, polished and shiny. She moves with ease and in due time. She stores all of the words, the intent, and the journey of my book in her shell. Lucy is equipped with shelves in her shell. I lovingly refer to them as her *shell shelves*. There, as if in a vault, the memoir was held with love until I was ready again to write. Thank you, Lucy.

The neat characteristics of tortoises are the following (these descriptions are taken from my friend and colleague Sarah Bamford Seidelmann's book *The Book of Beasties: Your A-to-Z Guide to the Illuminating Wisdom of Spirit Animals*):

The Tortoise:

- You are the happiest when you are unhurried.
- Vocation: The heavy shell of a tortoise naturally curbs its stride. Go slowly now, and do not push beyond a comfortable pace for yourself. And the "easy does it" attitude will get it all done.
- Root chakra: Always carrying their homes on their backs, tortoises are never without shelter. Light a candle and offer gratitude to your home today.
- Rest: Tortoises are known to rest up to sixteen hours a day. Schedule a day off when you can and have nourishing food prepared ahead of time. Take a nap, soak up the sun, journal.

Hmm, nothing there speaks to speed or quickness. Initially, I was a bit perplexed and befuddled with the tortoise as my book's spirit animal guide. Little did I know at that time how accurate the tortoise would prove to be. I was intently working from home, I felt very sheltered and covered as I ventured into business expansion with a strong vision and determination. I slept a lot. I took afternoons off. I started sometimes in the wee hours of the morning. And sometimes I just watched TV. It was quite an unusual schedule. And I was building my business. The business nearly doubled in that period and the infrastructure blossomed.

Returning now to focus on finishing writing my book, it feels as if I have not missed a beat in writing, nor have I lost any time. Truth be told, I feel right on time, which is both interesting and amazing.

As you lean into this book, know that I write this with the intention for you to learn my story, what makes me tick, and why I am so passionate about what I believe is my life's mission and work that yet remains to be accomplished. It is not a book to recruit you to my practice, my care, or my business, although I was counseled to have that be the focus. No, I do not agree with that. Nothing in my work is done without a clear intent and direction, so to write my story as an entrée to joining up is not in my DNA. And I've got the genomics report to prove it!

I write my story with the hopes that you get a glimpse into my life and, as you begin to know me, you see why my vision is important to patients, clients, and people in general. My various experiences, while unique to me, are a part of common humanity, meaning we all have something that has challenged us, moved us, and perhaps even nearly taken us out of this life. In my mind, resilience and lessons are the keys to standing, not even having to try and move forward. Sometimes just standing is okay.

Many people have told me that I hold a unique perspective on life. Perhaps that is true, and that is hard for me to know, because I live in my skin and in my experiences. While I certainly can empathize with others, I really only have walked in my own shoes.

Empathy is the ability to understand what others are feeling because you are in touch with what you are feeling. Erroneously, we think it means that we walk in another person's shoes. I am not sure that we can actually do that. But it sounds nice. However, I prefer empathy versus walking in another's shoes, because empathy means I am inhabiting myself and am in touch with myself, with good boundaries, so then I can be in touch with others. That seems more right to me.

We are all called to live a life of adventure and uniqueness. It is our choice if we follow through and live our lives in such a way. So many things, events, circumstances, and traumas can effectively "blow us out of the water." News flash: We are on a planet that is steeped in humanity and humanity's story. Mostly, the stories are dotted with trauma and difficulties. There are good parts too: happiness, love, contentment, triumphs, success, etc. This is not the planet of the blue, foamy drinks. I have been to that planet in my dreams, and for sure, it is not this planet that we are now on. Ahem.

No doubt, there are stories, and we all have them.

News flash (again): We are not our stories. Stories are what we have. Our stories do not define us unless we choose to let them. Our stories are what shape us, and our *choices* are how we discover how amazing we are and how stories are a part of our lives. We refer to this as *the story of our lives*. We are to live our lives, finding and understanding our stories while living our lives. There is a difference. And *choosing* to live our lives is where we begin.

Each of us is unique in our DNA, fingerprints, and views of the world. Even our stories are unique. Yet, they are not us, they are what happens to us. Our lives are what we do with our stories. We get to write the chapters and the endings, and all the while, we get to determine how we will live.

I love this quote from Brené Brown, which hangs in my office over my desk:

"Owning our story can be hard but not nearly as difficult as spending our lives running from it. Embracing our vulnerabilities is risky but not nearly as dangerous as giving up on love and belonging and joy—the experiences that make us the most vulnerable. Only when we are brave enough to explore the darkness will we discover the infinite power of our light."

May my story inspire you to know your own story and, more importantly, may you discover the infinite power of your light.

Chapter 1

The Accidental Shaman (Perhaps a Bit Reluctant Too)

"There are no accidents..."
—Robert H. Hopcke, Jungian psychologist and author of the 1997 national bestseller *There Are No Accidents: Synchronicity and the Stories of Our Lives*

"There are no accidents... there is only some purpose that we haven't yet understood."
—Deepak Chopra

"Nothing comes out of the blue."
—Sigmund Freud

"I think you are a shaman," said a friend. "What do you think?"

Hmm, I thought. I had not really ever given it too much consideration, other than when my husband Andy frequently introducing me to others as, "My wife, the witch doctor." *Eye roll.* Or when I would have an existential crisis and feel, deep in my bones, that I would probably have been burned at the stake in earlier times for the perspectives I hold as a physician. But, in my day-to-day life, being a shaman was not on my radar. Until it was. As I opened to the concept, more people began sharing their perspectives about why they felt that I was a shaman.

So, I looked into it.

The *Oxford English Dictionary* defines a shaman as: "a person regarded as having access to, and influence in, the world of good and evil spirits, and who practices magic or sorcery for the purpose of healing, divination, etc., typically by entering a trance state."

Okay, hmm. I had always connected the ideas of evil spirits, magic, or sorcery with not good things. *Are there other considerations*, I wondered?

What about the aspect of using shamanism for the purposes of healing? *Am I a healer?* That resonated. So I looked up *healer* in the *Oxford English Dictionary*. Here is what I found: "a person who seeks to cure diseases or heal injuries by means other than conventional medical treatment: *a spiritual healer and medium*; a person or thing that mends or repairs something; something that alleviates distress or anguish."

That for sure resonated with me. Then, looking at the etymology of the word *shaman*, I learned that it came from a combined German and Russian word dating back to 1689, as well as from multiple other northern European countries. And then in the Americas as well, in relation to the indigenous peoples. What stood out were the variations on the theme of the word—with slightly different cultural approaches in being a shaman, yet the roots of beliefs and roots of recovery for the individuals helped by shamans were similar.

Across the globe and for many, many years, healings, trances, potions (made from plants), and poultices, along with dances, songs, and deep seeing, listening, and intuition were the standard of care. Curious. I was practicing modern Western medicine, and yet I resonated strongly with those concepts, and my patients experienced outcomes that were not directly tied to a Western medical treatment plan. *Curious.*

In the book *The Hollow Bone*, by Colleen Deatsman, Sandra Ingerman, a well-known North American Shaman, says, "Shamanism is the oldest spiritual practice known to humankind. Many anthropologists have dated the practice back over 100,000 years, and it was and is practiced in every culture and the world over, and it survives in its many forms because it has been so successful at helping people and communities heal and stay whole." Ingerman continues, "Shamanism is a spiritual practice that is based on divine revelation, which means that we all can access spiritual knowledge to guide us in our lives and the times ahead. Shamanic practice requires no outside authorities, intermediaries, or even beliefs. Instead, shamanism provided a series of accessible tools that put you in contact with your deep inner knowing and spiritual allies that can help us, and at the same time, we can receive our own personal revelations that keep the work fresh and inspirited."

Ingerman said, "Shamanism is a way of life."

I was curious again: What are the chances that across the globe there is a commonality in our approaches to healing before we were ever considered a global community? Not an accident, in my humble opinion.

In further exploring Northern American shamanic works, I found a lot of practitioners using various integrative approaches, especially among the body workers, massage therapists, and people who hung their shingles out indicating that they were shamans. They brought their insights, skills, gifts, and trades to those who were suffering—and people received relief. Sometimes those healings occurred in spontaneous remissions of known medical conditions, and sometimes it was the suffering of the human soul that was liberated and healed. Either way, people did better, and their lives were transformed.

Also, sometimes, in my own practice, I've witnessed the opposite: shamanic healing, but not so much, with patients who found their way to my office and I helped them heal from not only their known diagnoses but also from their less-than-excellent experiences with non-licensed shamanic practitioners who were actually practicing medicine without a license. Sometimes, the attempts at cures were worse than what was originally ailing those patients.

Over time, for me, the concepts of shamanic work percolated deep into my soul and spirit. I mean, over years. What I am saying is that I did not declare myself a shaman after reading a few articles and books on shamanism. No, that was not what I did. In fact, I declined the invitations to shamanism and its implications, until I could no longer hold out. Even then, I did not announce it, as I had learned that those who self-declare as a shaman are probably not truly shamanic, but perhaps are appropriating aspects of healing modalities into other skills they have learned.

While often well-intended, such self-announced shamans may be helpful, but are perhaps not precise in their definition and standing. At times, I saw abuses within this concept of shamanism and its applications that left patients/people disillusioned and sometimes harmed. So I felt cautious, even while being a well-reputed physician, and perhaps because of being a well-reputed physician. I continued to be curious, even as I was not yet so convinced. Perhaps I did not want to out myself as a shaman. So I didn't. That is how I arrived and then sat for some time: I settled on the idea that I was both an accidental and reluctant shaman.

Accidental because I did not intend to become a shaman. *Reluctant*, because of what I just explained. However, I was still curious. So I leaned into the concept. I followed the tugging of my spirit and soul.

The tugging led me more toward the shamans in Europe and the United Kingdom, to the Celtic traditions in spirituality and religion. Even now, in recalling and writing about my initial exposure and considerations, I get goosebumps on my body. Something stirred deep within me that simply made sense. And it explained a lot of the experiences I have had with patients through the years. Patients would ask me, "How did you know that about me," or, "How did you know that is what I have?" I witnessed that time and time again. And people got better, were (dare I even say the word) cured. They were healed. The anguish of the soul, the pains of the body—both disappeared as our work together unfolded. Sometimes with medication, sometimes with hands-on treatments, such as osteopathy, and sometimes with supplements, lifestyle, and foods. But always through deep connection in what is called the *biofield*. This is the area of communication between the patient and me—an area of sacred space where symptoms, signs, and subjective ideas are held, and the place where the doctor and patient meet when in a therapeutic relationship.

Early on in my career, I learned that, for me, the doctor-patient relationship is sacred. Our communication was held in the highest regard, and the outcome unfolded based upon our shared experience. Yes, as the physician I may know more about medicine, clinical care, pathophysiology, etc., and the patient knows more about themselves (most of the time), but this is what I am talking about: the place where we go together to seek healing and understanding.

There is an amazing quote from the ancient Sufi poet and mystic Rumi:

"Out beyond ideas of wrongdoing and rightdoing,
There is a field. I'll meet you there."

Getting past judgment—of ourselves, our bodies, our illnesses, and our souls—allowed me to connect deeply with patients, sometimes with Western tools of medicine and sometimes with deep listening and reflection. All the while, patients simply got better.

Armed with that experience, understanding, and food for thought, there was nothing left to say other than: *This is me.* This is who I am and how I believe, love, live, and practice my craft of medicine.

I was a Shaman.

I have had all of the accouterments of modern medicine, licensing, board certifications (side note: I first typed "bard certifications," a Freudian slip when I meant "board certifications." A *bard* is a shamanic storyteller—LMAO. There are no accidents. Ya can't make this stuff up!) and now, at this stage of my career, some thirty-one years later, even the board certifications are ending as, clearly, the "bard certification" is becoming more evident and prominent in my work—the storytelling, narrative medicine, and the transferring of knowledge and wisdom by deep connection is the way I now practice. Sitting firmly outside of the insurances, having opted out of Medicare, I am now working one-on-one with patients in a direct-care model.

Yes, this is out there beyond the ideas of wrongdoing and rightdoing. This is truth-telling, without judgment: the healing of people and communities through a deep inner knowing, with spiritual allies and in a known lifestyle.

Yes, ladies and gentlemen, after thirty-one years as a traditional osteopathic physician, I can now proudly say, "I am a Shaman."

My Soul's Lesson

This quote from *The Hollow Bone* sums up my own experience of walking the shamanic path:

> "The shamanic path is the path of the heart and the soul. It is a path of beauty, wholeness, sacred living, oneness and connectedness with all things and non-things, awareness, mindfulness, respect, honor and gratitude. It's a path of extraordinary moments when Nature and Spirit speak more clearly than the racket of our mental chatter and we stop everything for that moment and take notice, listening and feeling the message."
>
> —Colleen Deatsman, *The Hollow Bone*

Chapter 2
Tire Swings and Lilacs

How do you like to go up in a swing,
Up in the air so blue?
Oh, I do think it the pleasantest thing
Ever a child can do!

Up in the air and over the wall,
Till I can see so wide,
River and trees and cattle and all
Over the countryside—

Till I look down on the garden green,
Down on the roof so brown—
Up in the air I go flying again,
Up in the air and down!

—Robert Louis Stevenson

Early Memories and Discovering Presence

Mom swung me and other kids in her arms between her legs until we were too big for her to swing us. As we swung, Mom would recite the Robert Louis Stevenson poem quoted above. That's a great memory. Mom was a real swinger, as many a kiddo was swung in her arms.

I remember my bedroom in our Fulton Street house in Grand Rapids, Michigan, as a place where I frequently escaped the crib and then could run around in a big circle through all of the rooms until I was captured and put back to bed. I remember watching Johnny Carson and *The Tonight Show*—that was always one of my favorite shows.

We had a landlady, Sokki, who lived in the backyard in a small house that felt very Hansel-and-Gretel-like to me. Inside Sokki's house, it was dark and smelled of cabbage. She had a very kind look in her eyes, I remember. My brother, who is two years older than me, would sit on Sokki's front stoop and declare quite boldly to the world, (actually, just to the neighborhood), "I hate home cooking." I am not sure that went over well with my mom. I do remember the situation, however...

Hackley Happiness

My mom told the story that while our new home on Hackley Street was being constructed, she had to "ride herd" on the builders. They often missed showing up on some days, claiming various reasons for not being on-site. But the more she persisted, the faster our home was built. She had a pretty good motive, as the current place we were living, on Fulton Street, would on occasion get infested. It was because the

Fulton Street house was next to a big commercial laundry facility. Apparently, one time, she went to flip up the collar on my jean jacket that I was wearing as a toddler and out popped a cockroach! She screamed bloody murder, but I don't remember that. Probably a good thing.

I also remember eating McDonald's lunch in the living room at the new house, while we sat on paint cans. Dad was painting the walls, and we were very soon to be moving in. Hamburgers were ten cents, and an orange drink was fifteen cents.

Ours was the second house constructed in the new neighborhood. I still have the blueprints, bill of sale, and mortgage coupon book my parents used to complete the project. I found those items when I was going through my mom's boxes that she left me after her passing. At the time I found the documents, Andy and I were constructing our current home, which was completed in 2021. Exploring the comparisons between the documents from 1965 and 2021 was fascinating. Their mortgage payment in 1965 was $73 a month; today, we pay a lot more!

I remember that the house, the yard, and the vastness of the back acres at the new house all felt like home to me, even when I was only three years old. I felt very connected to that home, yard, and "back forty."

Our backyard on Hackley Street extended into the woods and fields. Mom and Dad built us two tire swings on a huge old oak tree. My arms never could reach around that tree. That was our big-kids swing, when we no longer were swinging in mom's arm. We swung all year round, snow boots, leggings, and all.

The area directly behind our backyard went approximately a quarter mile east toward a two-lane road known as the East Beltline. North of our backyard however was a different story. That land went for miles. For me and the other kids in the neighborhood, that was our playground, our kingdom, our domain, our universe. We lived out there on the land during all seasons of the year. We went sledding in the winter, built forts in the summer, and hid out in the trees and the old dug-out foundation of what must have once been a homestead. The only limits were our imaginations.

As I grew up, my real freedom came from riding my bike almost anywhere that I could get permission to do so. In those days, if you had a bicycle, you were free. Anywhere your legs could take you, you went. Early morning swimming practice, basketball practice and, eventually, to work in Robinette's orchard. Towel wrapped around neck, swimsuit under my t-shirt and shorts, tennis shoes, and a water bottle. Life was good.

I also spent a considerable time dreaming about what I would do when I grew up. In my mind's eye, I always saw myself working at a desk. I pictured myself writing, reading, and making decisions.

The World Book Encyclopedia was wordy, but the *Childcraft* books that accompanied the encyclopedia were wonderful to read. There, I would get lost in the words on science, medicine, the healing of bones, and the like.

I was always curious about things and possessed a sense of wonder, which served to fuel my passion for exploration, learning, and adventure. That seemed very natural. I could sense an internal quest or calling that I always seemed to be responding to; it pulled me to go places and do something, either for real or in my mind and imagination. What I knew for sure was that it was a constant felt sense that I possessed —that I was born to live life, and I had some kind of purpose and reason for being. I saw life as an amazing adventure, with opportunities abounding everywhere I looked. "Doing that and going there" seemed like a good idea.

Foundations of a Felt Sense and Presence

Being outside was freedom, whether I was escaping from chores or simply being set free for the day. Either way, during all seasons, in all weather, I was outside. The big oak tree with its tire swings was my friend and playmate. I could go from tire swing to tire swing by pushing one tire swing real high and then jumping on the other to then meet in the middle and switch swings. Me, the tree, and the swings—what a combo. Sometimes I missed and landed in the soft sand beneath the tree. I felt connected to nature in a very strong way. When I felt connected to the earth, I also felt deeply connected to myself. I remember standing under the tree, feeling protected and cared for by its vastness.

In May each year, lilacs came in bloom. There was a grove of lilac bushes by the old homestead that was behind our yard. Each spring, I would go inside the grove and lie down on the ground. I would close my eyes and breathe in all the luscious scent of the lilacs. I remember not knowing where I ended and the lilacs began. I remember being in a meditative state, although that is not what I called it at that age. I just called it "getting lost in the lilacs."

Also, behind our garden was a field of tall grass and Queen Anne's lace flowers. That was a great place to rest in the heat of the day. There again, I would connect so strongly with nature that I had a felt sense of being one with the grass and flowers. My body felt connected, my soul felt whole, my spirit soared.

As I got older, and during the summer nights, I was allowed to sleep outside under the stars. I did that alone, sleeping on top of the picnic table, my sleeping bag wrapped under a tarp because of the dew. Watching the stars and listening to the chirping of crickets, feeling the gentle breeze, and smelling the outdoors settled my soul and quieted my spirit. Good thing I didn't toss and turn a lot!

I slept out on full moon nights and nights that were clear so I could watch the moon and the stars. Again, I had that same feeling of connection and being one with the sky and the universe itself. The feeling would go deep within me, into my soul and spirit. I felt held, comforted, and whole, while simply being connected to both nature and to myself.

My Soul's Lesson

Retrospectively, I have felt that very same felt sense of presence as an adult and recognized that it is what I have had all along. Many times, I wondered if I was connected, and if so, to what, or to whom. I wondered about God, Spirit, Love, Source and, throughout my life, I have experienced a variety of belief systems.

And then a lot of life happened. That always happens if you live long enough. Simply put, traumatic events happened to me, and then the trauma is what happens inside of us and as our body's response to the traumatic event. Being an earthly citizen and a part of common humanity, I know that each of us experiences traumatic events. And the body does register the trauma and keep the score. We wear our experiences and our physical body and our soul and spirit are scored with the score, as it were.

Dr. Gabor Maté, MD, teaches us that the primary thing we do as humans when we are traumatized is disconnect from ourselves. We have to, just to survive. We do this because we perceive it is not safe to stay connected. So we dissociate (the same thing as disconnecting). It's our rightful mechanism of adaptation and an appropriate nervous system response.

Then we are meant to reconnect by re-regulating. We are meant to go into the trauma response of fight, flight, freeze, or fawn, and then we come back to calmness. It is a human response, a mammalian response. Mostly, when trauma happens, we fail to re-connect or re-regulate. That is not a criticism; it is a fact of my experience with myself and with patients. This is a huge root cause of all chronic illness. Mine included.

Healing trauma is how we can reconnect to ourselves. When we are connected to ourselves, we can better connect with others. The safest place to be is connected to ourselves, and from there, we can go anywhere.

Learning this has helped me heal on so many levels. It is how I practice medicine. And it is the same way that I too have healed—physically, emotionally, and spiritually.

This is also how I discovered that I had shamanic tendencies. Experiencing a variety of situations that traumatized me, I learned that I was disconnected. I learned that I wanted to figure out my life, and I was bound and determined to do so, come hell or high water. Both hell and high water occurred: Hell was the various illnesses and griefs I experienced, and the high water was the seemingly never-ending stops and starts in my career. I often seemed close to what I felt I was supposed to be doing, but without ever quite landing or fully hitting the target. Experiencing that caused quite a bit of angst in my life and relationships. My physical body and emotions felt it too.

That may be a surprise to those who have known me for years. But, trust me, my innards and outers tell a different story. And that is just it: The body tells the story.

Listening to our body's wisdom sounds simple, perhaps trite; in actuality, it is profound and life-changing.

As I understood shamanism more, I learned that most of those traumatic events were considered either an initiation or attention-grabbing circumstance so that I would continue to pursue my spiritual path. As you will learn, there was a considerable length of time when I did not do that and, yes, there was hell to pay. It took a toll on my body, spirit, and soul.

I don't feel unique in that respect. I feel quite human, normal, and, as one could say, "You may not be good, but you are slow!" But even that is not true, really. I think I just had a lot of life lessons to learn. What is interesting is that when I would receive insight or guidance, even from people who did not know me, I was always encouraged to realize that I was right where I needed to be, even right on time, although, honestly, my progress felt like molasses in January. During the most anxious times, I felt certain that I was missing my life and missing my mark. Sometimes, I wanted to give up, to *never mind* about it. I am grateful that only lasted a bit, however. Now, some many moons later, I have the felt sense that it was all in divine timing and all in divine order. I couldn't be anywhere else than where I was, because, frankly, I was there, so I couldn't be anywhere else. If I were meant to be somewhere else, I would have been. Simplicity, but not simple.

So, without any further digressions, we can progress through the rest of this memoir knowing that, all along, I had a felt sense of presence, nature, being, and destiny. I am glad that I am sharing it with you now. Onward!

Chapter 3
First Loves and Grizzlies

"You are young, and the large world is yours. You are rich in seed and the earth must be kept fruitful. Cast your seed carefully, knowing that the world will be a better place with you in it."
—Author unknown

First loves could be defined, from a felt-sense perspective, as loves that are not only remembered but embodied. They are stored as sensations and meanings within us, waiting to be accessed and explored. These experiences are windows into the universal longing for connection, the sweetness of vulnerability, and the bittersweet beauty of emotional growth. Here are some of mine.

Basketball Is My Life—Jersey #22

Playing basketball was my life. It was my sport. My best friend, also named Mary, and I would play for hours. We each had basketball hoops in our driveways. In middle school, we played line basketball, which is where there are two teams lined up across from each other and then three players from each team play for the basket on either end of the floor. That was fun, but not enough action, because you had to pass the ball down the line and then the basketball went into action by the key. Not too much dribbling. I am not sure why that was a part of our physical education curriculum versus regular basketball, but in the end, it wasn't that bad, as I was on the fifth-grade and sixth-grade championship line basketball team.

Our middle school team played basketball in both the seventh and eighth grades, and there were tryouts and practices and the whole nine yards. By then, gone was the line to pass the ball down. It was full-on, dribble, pass, and shoot basketball.

Our biggest rivals were the teams from the other middle school, Hills and Dales, and St. Jude's, the local Catholic school. Both teams had good athletes. We always seemed to win, however. The good news about those rival teams was that by the time ninth grade rolled around, most of those girls came to the same public high school, so then we all got to play together.

Typically, my friend Mary and I would play all year 'round. It was our main activity besides schoolwork and chores. Our given basketball nicknames were Rip and Spaz, but I will not be taking any follow-up questions to that statement. Suffice to say, I was not Rip. Ahem.

Each summer, from eighth grade to twelfth grade, we practiced in our driveways. Both together and separately, we ran drills, played shooting games, and had free-throw contests, plus did a lot of one-on-one practice. Sinking shots from the edge of the driveway and keeping the basketball out of the street was key. At our house, I used the thirty-two-inch-wide brick wall between our two garage doors as a backstop for practicing my passes. For bounce passes, chest passes, overhead passes, and the like, the wall provided the needed feedback. Happily, I report, no windows or lights were broken, ever.

My dad added a concrete extension to the side of our driveway, giving us a whole lane to play in, and then some. We had a true free-throw line, so the layups and rebounding drills were easily completed. I brought out the kitchen timer and ran sprints and shuffle drills in a timed and measured fashion. Basketball was my world, and I loved it. In between my various chores and tasks, I would take breaks and go shoot hoops for ten or fifteen minutes, then go back inside to finish up. It broke up the monotony of dusting, for sure.

A Game for All Seasons

We played basketball in the cold weather too, sometimes. When needed, the driveway could be cleared of snow, and it was game on. Shooting from the snowbanks made for extra fun and they also provided a good stop for a runaway ball.

We had two basketballs. Mine was red, white, and blue, and my brothers' was red and white. You had to keep one basketball inside the house while playing in the cold because, in time, the cold would make the basketball stiff, so you had to trade it out for the warmed-up ball that had more bounce.

In the summers and on weekends, my uncles (my mom's brothers) came over and were keen on playing three-on-three, HORSE, and twenty-one in our driveway. We played for hours, and I loved it. Playing with the guys meant I had to up my game, as they were bigger and stronger than me. But that did not deter me. I wasn't intimidated.

We two Marys were inseparable regarding basketball, and together we attended summer basketball camps in western

Michigan, northern Michigan, and Indiana. And we practiced together. We lived about a mile apart and I rode my ten-speed bike to her house, pedaling fast with a basketball balanced on my hip all along the way. All of our practices and drills paid off when Mary and I both made the girls varsity basketball team as freshmen. We both started varsity basketball during our entire four-year high school careers. That was quite a thing. My other friend, Mary Ann (yes, there have been a lot of Marys in my life), designed a plaque that I hung on my bedroom wall that read: "Basketball is my life." Mary Ann painted it and stained it with a basketball. It had my jersey number, twenty-two, on it. That said it all.

High school sports and activities abounded, as I participated in marching band and even worked part-time throughout high school. Despite my lettering in multiple sports and participating in many activities, basketball was my first love.

Adulting with Choices

High school graduation loomed, and I was preparing for college, getting all of my ducks in a row for basketball, financial aid, and choosing a university to attend. As that progressed, life ended up taking a bigger turn than I had imagined.

In the fall of my senior year, one of my uncles (my mom's brother) moved from Michigan to Montana. It was a big deal to move, and there was a significant impact on my mom's life and her generation of family members, on my grandmother too. My uncle asked my dad to help with the move and, while unpacking in the small town in Montana, they eyed a bakery. My dad was trained as a baker, and he was a very good baker. However, during my senior year, he was not working very much, and it impacted our family. The family struggled because of his unemployment. At times throughout my parents' marriage, he struggled personally, the economy struggled, my parents struggled, and it seemed that life was very difficult for him. My brother and I often wondered why my parents stayed together and we felt that we would be supportive if they decided to divorce. My sister was quite young and, as she reports, she was blissfully unaware of the turmoil in the household. It turns out that my mom had a way of making things look just so. We witnessed Dad's difficulty in maintaining employment. While my parents were still together, they lived separately in the same household. Lots of eggshells were tread upon for many years, as it was a strained and challenging environment for us all.

In the spring of my senior year, my mom, grandma, and younger sister planned a trip to the town my uncle and his family had moved to in Montana. They were going on a spring break vacation to visit and see what this *Montana* was all about. My grandma kept asking, "What's Montana got that we don't got?"

A few days before they were to leave to go west, my uncle called my mom and dad in Michigan and informed my parents that the bakery was for sale. "Hey, Joe," he said, "you should jump on a plane and get out here. The guy wants to sell his bakery."

So my dad flew out a few days before my mom, grandma, and sister were scheduled to arrive as previously planned. That spontaneous trip led to my parents' decision to reconcile their relationship and move west from Michigan to Montana. That was settled—quickly, and without much ado. Apparently, my parents had a meeting of the minds while visiting Montana and sorted out their marriage and next steps in life.

Mind you, that was spring break of my senior year. In the

span of a few days, my parents reconciled and decided to move to Montana, buy a business, and sell our home in Michigan. They had never owned a business before. When they returned to Michigan after the Montana spring-break trip, they gave my brother, sister, and me the news. Decisions had been made. Then, as a family, we went about putting all of those steps in motion.

The remaining school year from April to June was completed and graduation occurred. My parents remained resolute with their decision to sell the house, move west, and work in a bakery. One day after my graduation open house, my dad, mom, younger sister, and I, along with a loaded moving truck, left Michigan for the Wild West.

My high school graduation open house in Michigan was held in our empty house. The only things left behind at Hackley Street were tire swings, lilacs, and a whole lot of wonderful memories of growing up while connecting with nature. For the open house, we had to get chairs and tables from the local fire department, where my dad was a volunteer, as all of our furniture and belongings were already packed in the moving truck. What started as a graduation open house turned into a huge send-off. Our friends and family gathered and said goodbye. It was a great party, and I was very excited to move.

New adventures. We're heading west! To Montana!
The mountains are calling, and I must go!

My whole family moved except for my older brother. He stayed in Michigan because he was enrolled at a local college and working; plus, by then, he was seriously dating my friend Mary Ann, so they were a "thing." Those crazy kids. They met, dated for nine years, and then WHAM, got married.

Such a thing, those two. I am happy to report however, that Joe and Mary Ann have had a great marriage, and they have given me three favorite nephews who were delightful as kiddos—and then even more joy and pride, as they are amazing men with their families.

Climb Every Mountain

Partway through my high school senior year, I decided to attend Northern Michigan University for college. NMU is in the Upper Peninsula of Michigan. I was going to play basketball there—well, at least try out for the team. I had already attended summer camps there and knew that NMU would be a good place to play and I could most likely continue with a basketball career. However, when the opportunity to move to Montana arose, I had to make a choice. I could stay in Michigan, go north to the Upper Peninsula for college, or I could move west with my parents and figure out college when I got there. While that did not necessarily mean I was not going to attend NMU, I saw that there were options—and the mountains were calling. They really felt like a tug on my heart, and I needed to answer. I needed to see what *that Montana* was all about. *And the mountains were calling*. I felt that in my soul. Deeply.

There were other times in my life when mountains tugged on my heart. In between my freshman and sophomore years, our band went to Austria to march and play in summer festivals. It was my first plane ride. Since watching *The Sound of Music* at age ten, I'd had a goal of visiting Austria and going to Salzburg to see all the *Sound of Music* sites. My dream came true in the summer of 1976. Most captivating was the feel of the mountains, how they were majestic and intimate at the same time. I was able to connect to the land by looking at and holding rocks, stones, and the branches of pine trees, and by smelling the fresh mountain air. Connection to nature and something much bigger than myself was easy for me to do, and Austria had the key elements—I was in love.

We landed in Munich and stayed in the Bavarian part of Germany, then went into Austria, still the Bavarian part of Austria, however. My connection to the country, mountains, people, nature, and pretty much everything was very strong. I could feel my whole body resonate strongly with that part of the world. It was so strong that I seriously considered moving to Austria and attending university there, just so I could live in the mountains and be a part of it all. I did not know the language, however, and, in the end, I think that is what changed my mind. But while I visited, I was in touch with my *felt sense* and desire to be in the mountains, in Bavaria, and connected to that part of the planet. I learned many years later that my DNA is 87% Bavarian German, so it makes great sense that I feel so much at home in that part of the world. (Don't ask me about my Neanderthal percentage; that is something I don't discuss, but it is there.)

Spring break vacations during my junior and senior years of high school were spent skiing in the Utah mountains. A lot of classmates went south to Florida; I went west to ski.

My aunt and cousin lived in Provo, Utah, and graciously allowed me and a friend to use their home as a base for spring skiing. OMG, the skiing was amazing. Both years provided excellent snow and experiences at all the major ski resorts: Snowbird, Alta, Park City, Park West, Sundance, Brighton, and Solitude. Some of those names have now changed, but what remained was my favorite resort in the whole world: Alta, Utah.

Alta had the ultimate powder, sunshine, and blue and blue/black runs. And then there was an amazing part of the mountain called The Ballroom, a huge bowl area that was wide and open and full of some of the best in-bounds powder skiing anywhere. I was in heaven and found that mountain skiing was another major love of my life.

I used to stand at the top of The Ballroom and, before I dropped down into it, say aloud, "My name is Mary Mark, and I ski!" That mountain salutation was taken directly from Olympic skier Jill Kinmont who, in 1955, tragically suffered a spinal cord injury at the same ski resort, Alta, but on a different part of the mountain. Reading her biography was inspiring, so much so that I went to our public library and researched her life, photocopied all of the articles, and hung copies of the magazine covers on my bedroom wall. The movie of her life was transformative. Beau Bridges played her boyfriend in the movie. Dreamy. So, when I skied Alta, I dreamed of my own *Mad Dick Buick* that I would one day meet.

That type of skiing in the mountains was such a great love for me. I felt so alive on the snow, making turns, skiing in powder, and carving my way down the whole mountain until my legs burned so badly I could hardly stand up. I felt free, alive, and connected to all the nature I could see and all the nature that was so much bigger than me. I often could not tell where the sense of myself ended and nature began. I was one with all of what was around me and it felt like a lightness of being on my insides. That was how connected I felt.

So, when the opportunity to move to Montana arose, I *had* to make the move with my parents and then sort out my life when I got there. What seemed both sudden and unexpected, and perhaps even confusing to others, felt so right, so clear and open, to me. The opportunity to be in the mountains could not compare with anything else for me. The mountains were calling—I had to go.

Those who had expected me to stay the course I had planned during my senior year and attend NMU in the Michigan Upper Peninsula sort of understood. For me, I saw only opportunity in moving west where it was wide open. My heart was fully connected with my decisions, and my body felt very good about the whole idea. Making decisions that way seemed very natural and appropriate for me.

Looking back, I see that type of patterned decision making as a way that I have always lived. Opportunities present themselves, plans are made, wheels set in motion, and then, if something arises, I take the opportunity to consider other options. I don't know if that is how most people are wired or not. What I do know is that my decision to entertain other opportunities does not arise from a fear of missing out, but rather from a place of curiosity, a place of being open to a variety of opportunities and experiences. When I evaluate opportunities, it's not that I just willy-nilly change my mind; it is more from the perspective that the new or other opportunity wasn't on the table at the time I made the other decisions. Therefore, I did not entertain the newer idea or option. But now that it is on the table, let's peek. Let's get curious and see what this could look like. Seems natural to me.

Hello, Mountains, It's Me, Mary

The drive west from Michigan to Montana took two very long days. A moving van can only go so fast, ya know. That meant we arrived in SW Montana well after dark. Frankly, it was the middle of the night. As we went over a mountain pass, we pulled the moving van and our truck (pulling a motorboat) into an overlook. Instead of looking down or out, we looked up. It was the first time I ever saw the Milky Way. *Amazing*. I was in tears, speechless, and did I mention *awestruck*. Not only for seeing the Milky Way but also—there were so many stars. I had never seen so many, ever. Goosebumps rise on my arms and neck even as I write this, from remembering such a felt sense of a welcome from our new home state and from the universe itself.

The very first morning I awoke in Montana, which was only a few wee hours after seeing the Milky Way, we headed up Mill Street to the "top of the mountain." We did not make it, because of snow that blocked the road, but I do remember the smells, sights, sounds, and feel of the mountain air. Again, that same felt sense of belonging washed over me and I knew I was home in my soul. We drove up in a yellow Chevy pick-up truck, the first of many trips "up Mill," as we called it, to Branham Lakes. I would tell people that at the end of our road was the top of a mountain! Yes, I used that as bragging rights!

Grizzlies and Quacks

A few weeks after arriving in Montana, I went on a tour of the University of Montana in Missoula. It was time to sort out my next steps for college. Would it be Northern Michigan or Montana? Both states had a lot to offer: excellent education and degree choices, the right size of the student population, sports, and nature.

There was a lot of nature around both universities. Montana had mountains and streams, Michigan had Lake Superior and the rugged "up north." What would probably be the deal-maker/breaker was tuition costs. I had just moved to Montana, but I had all of my financial aid set for NMU and was considered an in-state resident there. For UM, I had not even applied for admission or financial aid yet. Yikes.

But then a door opened. In a meeting at the registrar's office at UM, they informed me that because my parents owned a business in Montana, I was considered an in-state student for tuition costs! What?! Say *what*?! With me in that meeting were a couple of newly made girlfriends from the town we had just moved to who were also cementing their enrollment at UM. When I replied to the administrator that my parents had only lived in the state for about three weeks, I got punched in the arm by one of my new friends, who gave me "the look." I did not say anything more. I was *in*... in-state!

That settled it. I was going to the University of Montana in Missoula, Montana. I was going to be a Grizzly! Go Griz!

Students were assigned advisors in college. I met with a very nice professor in the Forestry building. Still attracted to those trees! He was in the sciences and his office was in the Forestry building. After a brief discussion and such (there may have been a questionnaire; I don't recall), he declared, "You should be an osteopathic physician." I promptly replied, "Um, I don't think so. They are quacks!" That was a very deep, visceral response to a seemingly appropriate conclusion by that professor. And, yes, there is a story here. It is a difficult one, however, but, again, that is another first love of mine.

Nature and Its Ways—A Felt Sense of Love and Loss

One of my mom's brothers (my mom had five brothers) married a very nice lady, and together they worked at a nature center in our city in Michigan, before I moved to Montana. Part of their work was through the public school system and part was through a museum. In the summers, I took classes at the nature center. I think I may have been allowed to attend a year earlier than the usual age limit, because of my connections. That was great, fine by me. I was all-in for the nature classes, including entomology, ornithology, and Pioneer Ways (bugs, birds, and pioneers). I was in heaven.

My aunt was my instructor for a couple of classes. We were attached at the hip (I thought so, anyway). My aunt was very, *very* smart, very quiet, and an amazingly patient teacher. She was my idol. I wanted to grow up and know everything she knew. I wanted to wear blue jeans and a bandana on my head, just like her. Mainly, I wanted to be in nature with her all the time.

During the outdoor classes, I sat next to her in the field identifying meadowlarks, robins, and bluebirds by their colors, flights, and songs. Bugs were another thing. We had to capture them and then euthanize them with our glass jars and acetone. And then, before the rigor set in, mount them carefully in a very insect-looking manner, with pins. Small confession: I used tools and rarely touched the insects, dead or alive. But still, my insect taxidermy, known as *pinning* or *mounting*, turned out pretty good (no stuffing required).

Pioneer class was a tremendous learning experience. Really, it was my first exposure to herbs and organic gardening. We used marigolds as insect-repellent plants by the vegetables, and harvested sumac berries to make sumac-aid, or sumac-lemonade. It was delicious. We also made soap, beeswax candles, and—drumroll, please—sassafras tea. It tasted like licorice. *Yum*!

It made sense to work in harmony with the earth, to use the plants to help support and protect other plants. It made sense that they worked together and that we too should work in harmony using ingredients from the earth, like beeswax for candles, lye and ash for soap. It all deeply resonated with me.

As happy as those memories are, difficulty—rather disaster and tragedy—came shortly thereafter. My aunt required surgery for a routine issue (if there is such a thing) and suffered a medical complication and lost her life. She passed away the summer between my seventh and eighth grades. It was later in the summer, near my birthday. We gathered flowers from the fields around our house, bouquet upon bouquet of daisies, black-eyed Susans, and Queen Anne's lace. A bower for her funeral.

We were all were heartbroken. We were confused. We were bewildered. We were in agony. Losing my aunt was one of the first major losses in my life—a first love, lost. I didn't understand, but deep in my gut something, wasn't right about the explanations given by the physicians, the osteopathic physicians. It simply did not add up. It did not make sense. And she was gone.

It would be many years before I learned what caused the death of my aunt. Intuitively, all along I felt something wasn't right about the explanations, and I was right. But it was there, in that circumstance, that I learned from my family that osteopaths are quacks. Hence, my bias was well-formed. It seemed reasonable. Until it wasn't. That too took time to unfold, but during my years at the University of Montana, I did not pursue becoming an osteopath.

University life was the life for me! Studying hard, playing hard, making new friends, and being on my own—it all suited me quite well. My mom and sister moved me into the all-female dorm Corbin-Brantley Hall. Room 350. It overlooked the courtyard and grass that would come to be known as *Brantley beach*, a place to sunbathe, play frisbee, and drink Rainier beer. Those days were short-lived, at least the Rainier beer days, because of another big change that my life was going to take. But first, let's get to the basketball part of college.

Basketball and Life Diverge

Having switched universities, I left behind connections and solid opportunities to play basketball at NMU back in Michigan. I thought it would be easy to introduce myself to the University of Montana women's basketball coach and then try out for the team. That was pretty much how it was across colleges at that time. Who knew that UM would be ahead of their time. And that I was behind the times. *Ugh.*

The Lady Griz, as they were called, was a burgeoning program gaining momentum in the Big Sky Conference. It was that year, my freshman year, that the coach decided that in order to be able to play for the Lady Griz, and even try out for the Lady Griz, you had to be invited. It was called *closed tryouts.* I wasn't invited, only because I wasn't heard of. I was a walk-on, had just moved from Michigan, and the coach did not know who I was.

You can't really fault a gal for moving across the country and deciding to change universities, can you? That was unfortunately not the point. As it was, the coach decided to let me work out with the team, because I really was persistent in my request and because they also had a JV team. While they only practiced and there were no official games, if I got on the JV team, I could at least play basketball with others. So, for a week, I worked out with the Lady Griz, the athletes who were invited to try out and those who were already on the team.

At the end of the week, Coach Selvig and I had another discussion, one of the hardest of my young life. He said that I played very well, had good skills and basketball sense, and that I would have made the Lady Griz squad had I been invited. He also said that I could be a player on the JV team, but he had to stick to his original plan of the closed try-outs. I was out and, therefore, I was not able to continue my basketball career after high school, despite the talent, dedication, and drive to do so. One of my first loves ended abruptly. I was heartbroken. It was gut-wrenching, agonizing, and maddening all at the same time. Another first love lost.

How do you resolve feelings like this at that age? I did not, initially, nor for quite some time. I buried my grief, disappointment, and sadness and tried to rationalize that there was more to life than basketball, that life would go on; but I still had the plaque that said basketball was my life. It was pure anguish and disappointment. I did not want to leave the University of Montana, because I loved the campus already and felt very connected to it, but I felt adrift in my soul. Basketball was such a part of my life, and that chapter seemed to be having a firm closure. A final buzzer, if you will.

Finding Meaning with a Couple of Gotchas

There were other times in my college career when regret and bittersweet feelings would surface as well. It was clear then that I hadn't fully healed from the felt sense of rejection by Coach Selvig.

I made friends with some of the Lady Griz, as we had classes together in the PE department. Others could not make sense of the coach's decision either, especially when we were all together in the basketball activity class. I played as well as any of the team players. We all agreed, it was kinda weird. A small bit of "gotcha" came about too, when we were in refereeing class together and I called a tight game on all those Lady Griz—no three seconds in the lane was allowed, *ever!*

My degree choice was in athletic training, so that meant in the final two years, I directly cared for athletes and assisted at various athletic events, and that included the Lady Griz basketball team. As a result, I saw life from both sides during those games, seasons, and years. Bittersweet feelings lingered my entire time at UM. Those feelings did not interfere with my learning, or with my work with the athletes. In fact, they kinda spurred me on.

I became very determined the last two years of my undergraduate studies. I wanted to excel because I was still around and maybe even remind folks of what they missed out on, perhaps. But, more than that, I wanted to apply to graduate schools for athletic training. It was clear that a master's degree was required for the best career opportunities, and so I wanted to go to the best master's program available. There were three universities that were tops for master's degrees in athletic training: University of Virginia, Arizona State, and Michigan State. Any one of those universities were fair game, and it was game-on to get accepted.

At the University of Montana, my athletic training degree came through the School of Education and Montana had one of the premiere programs in the nation. Who knew? I did not know that when I matriculated there. So, in the end, getting an excellent education and having exposure to athletes and competition came in handy for the next stages of my career and life.

I also made a lifelong friend as a result of attending UM: Jill. I met her on her wedding day, held her babies, and then, many years later, she was in my wedding. That friendship remains a great part of my life.

My Soul's Lesson

Early life brought first loves and subsequent losses of some of my first loves. All were monumental, all were life-changing. It would take some time and then a "somewhere down the road" kind of insight, awareness, and resolution before I was helped with the grief of those losses. I think that is sometimes how life is. We don't always have access to the whys, even if we are curious. Life can move along in mysterious ways.

What is true is that I did not ever give up. I kept looking for the next steps, I resolved as many feelings and connections I could, as well as experimented with a lot of different aspects of life. I was very much in love with life and relished the many opportunities I was fortunate to explore.

I guess, in many ways, I had several first loves. And when the losses came, I chose how I wanted to respond. I dug in and found more opportunities, leaving behind the grief. Not necessarily processing or experiencing the grief, but leaving the experiences behind. What I did not realize at the time was how such experiences can accumulate over time and have influence on our perspectives.

What I know for sure is that all of those events—the moves, changing universities, and every single love and loss of love—has made me the person I am today. I have great memories of my years as a Griz and my university experiences. I am grateful for every single thing I experienced, my friendships, degree choices, and how well the UM prepared me for life. So, to be clear, I did not pursue medicine while in my undergraduate program. But, just in case, I did take nearly all of the premed courses, and my degree in athletic training afforded me a foot in the door for musculoskeletal medicine. As it turns out, that is one of the fundamentals of osteopathic medicine. Curious. Interesting.

After being accepted into both the University of Virginia program and Michigan State program, I chose to pursue my master's degree at MSU, for two reasons: It was my home state and I had a lot of family there, and one of my main instructors from UM also had attended MSU and highly recommended it. What I was to find out later, in a twist of life, was that Michigan State University was also the home of the College of Osteopathic Medicine, one of the leading osteopathic colleges in the nation. Who knew? I certainly did not know that. Curious. Interesting.

Now that I am in the advice-giving business and I get paid for my opinions, I know how it is when you know that what you are sharing with someone is "gold" for them, and yet the advice is rejected, like when I initially rejected the professor's suggestion that I study to become an osteopathic physician. Ugh... yet quiet hope hangs in the air.

As it worked out, for me, in time and after part of graduate school, osteopathic medicine became another first love experience. I always wanted, deep down on the inside, to be a doctor. Always. It was a first love from very early on. Basketball, nature classes, grief and loss, moving to the mountains, becoming a Grizzly, and thinking osteopathic physicians were quacks were all part of that journey—my life's journey of a full education and a set of life experiences of first loves and first loves lost.

I wish I could remember the name of my advisor who suggested osteopathic medicine, and I often wonder if he is still alive. Perhaps so. Upon reflection, I am grateful for his insight, for his directive and advice. He remained resolute with his advice every time we met. Even though my position, to his knowledge, never changed.

Often, when outside under the sky, the big sky, I have raised my hands and offered up a prayer of thanksgiving for my advisor and his sage advice that stood the test of time. *Thank you, thank you. Amen.*

Chapter 4
Parents and Elders—Both Are Difficult to Raise

"The light you give off.
did not come from a pelvis.
Your features did not begin in semen.
Don't try to hide inside anger,
radiance that cannot be hidden."
—Rumi

"I am not going to negotiate who I am with you, because then I may fit in with you, but I no longer belong to myself. I will not betray myself in order to belong."
—Brené Brown

"You belong everywhere and nowhere."
—Maya Angelou

Adulting As I learned It

As I understand it, the whole goal of parenting is to raise decent, respectful, law-abiding, independent children to become good adults. The verb is *adulting*. This is my understanding from only one side of the equation, as I do not have any living children. I am a proud dog-mom, and I am convinced our labradoodle is a good canine citizen, along with being quite a character who is totally embodied and full of life.

That being said, I also believe that we choose our parents. This is an existential statement that I literally have no proof about, but it is my belief. Once I settled on that belief, my entire nervous system relaxed, and I no longer fought to either get out of my family or to stay in my family. I settled in and learned from those around me, and I worked on being the best "me" for them as well.

In a mystical sense, I believed we all were placed together for our mutual benefit, in that we are all in a universe that is both kind and benevolent. And then there is the DNA, which really is the icing on the cake as to how much DNA a nuclear family shares, coupled with pretty much the same sets of values and nurturing—yet we are all so individual and so unique. I have often wondered, in response to my siblings' bewilderment of me, if we actually all three came from the same womb! My mother assured me that we did.

Developmental psychology, early education, school clubs, 4-H, Girl Scouts and Boy Scouts, and many other organizations are geared toward successful social and educational growth of children, directly and indirectly. Again, the goal is adulting.

The research shows that a solid home base is also important. We are coming into greater and greater understanding regarding adverse childhood events (ACEs) and how they contribute to social determinants of health. Literally, this is a public health issue that contributes to early chronic disease onset, delayed skills, and challenges with entering the workforce. If we closely examine this topic, we could say that, in our current culture and climate, this topic and its fall-out is near epidemic in its proportion. Adulting is a thing, and there are so many ways we need to adjust our teaching, medical care, parenting, and skills-building in order to help young people to adult.

I had good parents, and they were complicated. They often did not understand me or, more accurately, they thought they understood me, but they really just pigeon-holed me and thought I was up to something. The truth is that I am wired for curiosity, exploration, innovation, and change. So it was hard for them to stay ahead of me, and certainly much harder to control me. There were a lot of struggles outwardly and inwardly when I was growing up. And there was some generational trauma that I experienced from both parents. They each had traumatic upbringings. That is not unique; rather, it is part of the human condition. There are specifics to each of us that allow our growing up experience to be unique.

Also, I was involved in religious organizations steeped in shepherding doctrine and purity movements that were so restrictive and legalistic that I fought and resisted on the inside just to survive. It took a toll on my physical, mental, and spiritual health.

At a very young age (I think it's even how I came into the world), I was comfortable with myself—until I wasn't. Early on, I had a sense of style, perspective, and a certain beingness that I could feel. I remember exploring outside with curiosity and some trepidation about being too far away, but I was always curious about what the world held for me. I believe I was meant to live a full and exciting life. I still believe—despite life and its various twists and turns—that we live in a friendly universe, and we learn to navigate life through our various experiences as adults.

Think about it. Childhood is eighteen years, give or take, and our adult years are anywhere from fifty to seventy-plus years. So, I am curious about why we are so focused on what our childhoods were all about. I am sure there are scholars who are rolling their eyes at that idea, but it strikes me that if we focus only on our childhoods while we are adults, we may potentially miss what is going on right in front of us.

To be sure, I encourage each of us to sort out our childhoods, to make sense of what happened and understand and repair various unhealthy patterns and traumatic events. We need not carry all of our childhood issues into adulthood. In fact, it is healthier to not do that. There are so many resources available to use today that did not exist when I was a youngster. So, my advice to you is that you make sure you all get that stuff sorted. You're welcome.

In the ceremonies chapter coming up, I write about ceremony number one and number two. The space between them is twenty-two years. So much of life happened in that time span. It was recently suggested to me that most likely all the major trauma in my life happened before the first ceremony, so up through to 2002. When I left the church in 2002, I was done, and we were also striking out as a new family to Colorado and, essentially, at some level we were adulting as a family. For much of the time, in the twenty-two years between ceremonies one and two, I was in a fight, flight, freeze, or fawn pattern. Those are the four trauma patterns that are driven by our autonomic nervous system, which is inextricably linked to our mental health and our hormonal and immunological systems (psycho-neuro-endo-immune system). When I work with patients and am providing trauma-informed care, I talk about those as the four food groups of trauma. Ha. Sometimes it helps to lighten the discussion, leaning on laughter as the best medicine.

In 2002, when I left the church and baby-bathwatered that whole scene, I decided to never again negotiate who I was, and accepted that I most likely would not truly belong anywhere again. In fact, I knew I would not seek out any religious community to commit to again. I was my own person. That has remained true to this writing. I do not suspect that perspective will change. That arose from the twenty-two years I rotated strongly through the fight, flight, freeze, fawn trauma responses like clockwork.

As I said, my parents were complicated. I loved my mom and my dad deeply, completely. And I learned they were human. We had seasons of good and bad times. My parents were married for thirty-one years. During the last years, my dad made a choice to leave our family and move to a different part of Montana to live with a different woman and her family. It's true that my dad left my mom, but the full truth is that when my mom confronted my dad about his abandonment, he said that he was leaving not only her, but the whole family. Granted, in conversations like that, we may expect a person to speak out of spite with the intention of causing hurt, and that probably was true, but the actions of my father to further stay estranged and separate from his three children reinforced his statement, and thus he was essentially estranged from us for almost the next thirty-one years.

I don't understand his actions, not from him as a father or

a husband. However, I will stay in the lane I'm writing this from: a daughter's perspective. In writing this, I will shield certain events, out of respect for my father's life and journey. The same is true for my mom. What I can say is that I observed patterns in their relationship when I was growing up, and then patterns in the whole family. Those made deep impressions upon my psyche. As I grew to understand trauma-informed care as a physician, I gained a better understanding of my parents' humanness, and the events that we would consider adverse childhood experiences that contributed to their lifelong struggles.

Shortly before my dad passed over in 2018, I was able to make sense of my dad's childhood experiences and I was able to talk with my mom about them. My father's traumas stemmed from growing up attending a parochial school and living in a Catholic community. I recall that after I shared all of my theories and insights about my dad's early traumas and how they then played out in his life and thus their marriage, Mom was quiet for a few moments. I could see that she was scrolling back through the thirty-one years with my Dad and cataloging the various events that stood out to her from our conversation. Then she slowly said, "Well, now my entire marriage makes sense." Knowing my mom understood there had been trauma as an experience framework for my dad was such a breakthrough for her, a true healing, a release.

Before my dad's passing, my mom was able to write to my dad and forgive him, which is something that she had sworn she would never do. Point of fact, that struggle for her was such a significant part of her life's journey that when she resolved all of those feelings and arrived at forgiveness, I wondered if she felt it was then okay for her to be done with life too. I will never know for sure, but she did pass away about four months after my father passed, and her death was unexpected.

The Elders as Trusted Others

The elders are the church leaders that I encountered during my stint as a Pentecostal and Evangelical. Those years were between 1980 and 2002. Twenty-two years. Hmm, I just realized that the time before ceremony one was twenty-two years and the time in between ceremonies one and two was twenty-two years (I will tell you about those ceremonies in upcoming chapters). Interesting. Curious.

Longing for Belonging

As a young adult and into adulthood, I was continually held with both doubt and suspicion for what my intentions and actions were. I was perceived as different, misunderstood. Certainly, one to watch out for. I was labeled as rebellious, independent, and strong-minded. There was always something in me the leadership in many positions could not put their finger on that seemed "off" to them.

That message came through loud and clear in the religious communities I belonged to. While I was raised Catholic, I was "born again" in my freshman year of college into the Pentecostal church. Then, while attending graduate and medical schools at Michigan State University, I was a part of Maranatha Campus Ministries, which turned out to be pretty much a cult community. That fact I was unaware of at the time, however.

The pressure on me regarding my own ambiguity about family life, career, and next steps caused me a great deal of anxiety, but moreover a great deal of self-doubt. While I was adulting in my life, my parents were separated, and things were getting messy with them. My mom was struggling, and it put a lot of pressure on me. There wasn't anywhere to turn except to the religious community that I was a part of. There, the leaders felt ambiguous about me because I was, well, I was me. When the leaders came to me and said things like, "You have a lot of potential, but just not now," I felt torn on the inside about what my life could or should look like. I did not know where to turn, where I could go next, or how to feel safe.

Work and studying had always been an anchor for me, so I continued with my graduate work, seriously considered medical school, and worked at a physical therapy clinic. I mentioned already that I always wanted to be a doctor. I loved the white coat, the smell of antiseptic, and scrubbing my hands clean like I was a surgeon. I read about science, anatomy, and physiology, I had loved my undergraduate degree work and wanted more. I wanted to be unrestricted in what my work could be, so that meant I needed to be a physician, as that would allow for the most license to be what and who I wanted to be.

In the religious communities I belonged to, it seemed that I was presented with a choice between either a career in medicine or being an ideal wife, mother, and helper in the church. What came through was that God loved me and had a wonderful plan for my life and, "We, as your church elders, know what is best for you."

The Trusted Others

That conflict created suffering in my soul and was felt as a difficulty to stay connected inside of me. I felt fractured in my soul and body and spirit because I was being told not to trust myself or my thoughts, but to trust others who instructed me that *they had my best interests at heart.* At the time, I did not understand the implications of this tension in my body and soul. I did not know that it contributed greatly to illness because it was clearly taking me out of my ease and placing me in dis-ease, *disease.*

I bent to the wishes and requests of others, at the expense of following my own soul and its knowing of my own way forward. What always seemed to happen was that my way was not the religious community's way and, therefore, it was not God's way. That was why I was told I was always a contrarian and rebellious—because I held fast to what I felt I wanted and what I was sensing for my life, and it was not in keeping with the religious expectations of my elders. I was fulfilling and adhering to a learned or cultured adaptation that is called *socialization.* What I wanted was acceptance and belonging, which meant not pursuing becoming a physician; and what my soul wanted was for me to be a physician. That my soul was at odds with the leaders and what they thought was good for me caused the internal tension, anxiety, and dysregulation of my neuro-endo-immune system. I was fighting on the inside and it was disrupting my health. So, for a while, I worked on my master's degree and got a full-time job in a physical therapy clinic that allowed me to further develop my skills in musculoskeletal treatment. Work had always been a good way for me to sort things out. It kept me occupied. I was productive, curious, and wanted to stay busy —and I was supporting myself as a young adult.

What's odd is that, during that time, my professional skills increased greatly. That ran in tandem with my desire to become a physician, which continued to grow, and the resistance of the elders toward me increased as well. That tension, that environment, that... pulling on my soul, created more stress in me. I wanted to be accepted and I wanted to conform to what others wanted for me—that rose out of a deep desire to belong. I wanted to be obedient to God's will. I wanted to be accepted by God and not seen as rebellious. The bending one's soul to fit into someone else's ideas is the definition of cultural conditioning. I negotiated myself away in order to belong. When I heard what the trusted others had to say about my best interests, it did not resonate with my soul. Yet I wanted to belong. I did not want to be rejected.

Rejection was an issue I was experiencing with my own family, primarily my parents. During that season in life, my parents were struggling and ending their marriage. It was difficult and traumatic, for them and for me as one of their children. I experienced the trauma from my parents' marriage disintegrating as rejection from my biological family. Both parents were difficult to deal with because of their own issues, choices, and the trauma they experienced and caused. At that same time, I did not want to experience rejection from my religious family. Not fitting in, not belonging to God, was a pain that I could not endure. That created a significant response within my body, a trauma response, and it made me susceptible to illness because of the dis-ease. What I did not realize at the time was that it also was the roots of what healers call *shaman sickness* or *healer's syndrome*.

> "Health challenges caused by illness, injuries and accidents—often severe and considered untreatable—are common life-crisis callings. This kind of calling involves a devastating decline in health and often a feeling of imminent death or a near-death experience.

Shamans who have these experiences are considered wounded healers."
—Colleen Deatsman

What the trusted others thought about me caused me to feel small, threatened, ashamed, and marginalized. I was told that I could not—moreover, should not—trust myself, my internal guidance. The soul was "the flesh"—corrupt, sinful, and full of evil. Instead, I needed to put all of my trust in God and in what others felt was right for me.

To do that is to create what is known as an *external locus of control*. This means that control stems from external forces. You believe that events outside of your control drive your actions and the outcomes you get. In that situation, you do what others think best for you, rather than following your own soul or heart. Knowingly, or most often unknowingly, you trade your authenticity, your agency, for acceptance and belonging. I did that in those circumstances.

In both of those arenas, acceptance and belonging, I was told to place my trust outside of me: outside of my control, outside of my being and beingness. The external locus of control was giving myself over to the will of God and to what others understood the will of God for me to be. On the inside of me however, it felt divisive, confusing, and confounding to my soul. I was not at peace, although I belonged. I was not trusting myself, but I was being trusted by the trusted others. That meant I was accepted, and I was a part of something, but I wasn't authentic, because of my internal struggle and loss of my internal locus of control. That was the whole thing: Give up control, let God control, and we will tell you what you are meant to do and be and become. That combination and control were at the roots of my anxiety and self-doubt, which I had for many years.

While I was told not to trust my thoughts, my body, or what my desires were—because they ran contrary to the will of God—I saw others doing what they felt were their heart's desire and being allowed, encouraged, and released into for their lives, their gifts, and callings in various aspects of ministry, college life, dating, marriage, and next steps. All the while, I was told to wait. That did not make sense to me.

What I don't know, but would consider retrospectively to be the case, is that the folks who were seemingly following their heart's desire, the same ones who were in leadership, ministry, and other more visible positions, did that while also possibly losing their authenticity. Did they give themselves over to what others thought best for them? Did they live their lives by an external locus of control? Did they also gain acceptance by receiving the permission of the trusted others versus following their soul's guidance? Perhaps, but I cannot say.

Graduate School and Mononucleosis

During that time, I was enrolled in graduate school at Michigan State, studying athletic training and spinal biomechanics. As mentioned, I was also trying to fit into a campus ministry, which was not really going well. I wanted to fit in, badly. I wanted to be accepted, badly, I wanted to do the "will of God," badly. My experience, however, was "badly." Being a young woman of ambition, goals, and focus, I was told that I needed to be broken down before God would build me up. I was told that I did not fit because I was too independent-thinking and "rebellious." They even used a nursery rhyme: "Mary, Mary, quite contrary."

In actuality, I was not contrary, I just had my own way of seeing things. While that was not new to me, it was to them and, apparently, it was perceived as a threat. Not only was I told that I did not fit, I was also told that I was not a Christian, I was not a believer. Apparently, I had received a false conversion and needed to get saved again. Then baptized again. And again. All told, I was saved three times and baptized four times (including the infant Catholic baptism, which I recognized, but the campus ministry did not recognize).

As that was going on, a couple of years passed and I became quite ill with mononucleosis, chronic fatigue, and fibromyalgia. I was even checked multiple times for Hodgkin's lymphoma, which, thankfully, I did not have. But I became very ill. I had to drop out of graduate school because I could barely function. I had found employment, which was great, but to attempt both to work full-time and attend graduate school full-time was too much physically. It was also too much emotionally and spiritually. Yet I trudged onward, wanting desperately to fit in, to not be rejected. I received IV antibiotics and gamma globulin daily for weeks, as I couldn't kick round-robin infections of strep, pseudomonas, and Epstein-Barr virus. I was one sick pup, missing weeks of work and graduate classes.

My soul wanted to follow the destiny on my life, and the trusted others had a lot to say about what that should look like, which did not resonate with me. Instead, I had a felt sense that I was still waiting for my life to begin, but I wasn't sure as to why or what I was waiting for. Life, God, my destiny, my holy calling? What was I waiting for? What was going on? I was told by the trusted others to be patient and continue to serve.

Medical School Was My Soul's Desire

What became clear, crystal clear, was that the *only* thing I wanted to be was a doctor, an osteopathic physician. That's it.

I longed for it, like the breath it took to live. I had to become a physician.

As I was finishing some of my master's programs in spinal biomechanics, I decided to apply to medical school at Michigan State University and another university in Texas. As mentioned, I was ill with mono, chronic fatigue, and fibromyalgia. By then, that also meant I was a spiritual failure, as it appeared that I did not have the faith to get better (or I would have already), and to take on any type of life change other than working and serving in the church was not God's will—more like my own pride and ambition. Those were the wise words of the trusted others. Even writing this now leads to a felt sense of sadness and a deep well of self-compassion, because of the spiritual wounding that occurred back then. It was a moral injury done in the name of religion. Not cool. Not cool.

The first time I applied to medical school, I still was fully ill with mono and chronic fatigue syndrome. I did not get accepted into either medical school. I was disappointed but not detoured. There was always next year.

During that time, I worked in a physical therapy clinic. I had an awesome boss who was both fair and honest. His guidance spurred a lot of much-needed and appreciated growth in my life. It also solidified my soul's desire for medicine. *I had to be a doctor—there simply was nothing else to be, nothing else to do.*

I practiced on patients in the physical therapy clinic. I had a newly released textbook on osteopathic manipulation, by Dr. Phil Greenman (a man who would later become a mentor). When evaluating patients, I followed the osteopathic evaluation method and applied treatments, the patients got well, quickly. OMG... I was on to something, and certainly in my element! That success accompanied a felt sense of well-being.

The more I studied osteopathic manipulation treatments, the better my health got, the happier I became, and the fuller my soul felt. Fitting in began to look like being myself and bringing healing to my patients.

One Less Organ in This Person

Wanting to apply to medical school again the next year, I had to get fully well, and that meant considering a tonsillectomy. I kept having recurring strep infections and I lived on antibiotics. So, as an adult (not for the faint of heart), I had a tonsillectomy—proof that it is easier to have that surgery as a child and have all the ice cream you want. As an adult, however, it was a challenge to recover. While there were no complications, it did take a full three weeks to return to work and be on the mend. The surgeon confirmed the chronically infected tonsils and said it was one of the worst cases he had ever seen.

Post-tonsillectomy—and having applied to and been accepted into only one medical school, Michigan State University College of Osteopathic Medicine—I began my journey of becoming a physician, my soul's desire and what felt like my true calling. That was, however, much to the chagrin of the trusted others.

The Two Shall Become One

After residency and a couple of years in practice, it felt like the timing was right. I was ready. So, one day during a prayer meeting, I called in a husband. Some may call it manifesting. I put a timeframe out there during prayer to meet and enter a serious relationship within the next nine months. This is a true story. It was shortly after that prayer meeting that Andy came into our local church from an ad in the newspaper. The local church ran a summer special of six or seven advertisements in *The Grand Rapids Press.* Andy saw the ad and began attending our church. It would be a few months until we formally met, but it seems reasonable that I called him in, so to speak. All things considered, doing so seemed like a good way to get things started.

Andy and I met, started dating, became engaged, and married, all within a five-month span. It is said that when you know, you know. That was true for us. The whole process took just about nine months, give or take a couple of weeks. Not bad for timing.

Andy and I had discussed that, most likely, our marriage would lead us to relocate to a larger city, due to the nature of Andy's career. As an electrical engineer, he wrote code for pretty sophisticated projects, and there were certain cities in the USA that had a lot more to offer for career opportunities than West Michigan.

When the time came, and with very good intentions, we relocated from West Michigan to the West, to Colorado, to be specific. We have moved a few times since then, each time for our work and various career opportunities. Some opportunities were better than others. But we always felt that no matter where we were or how things were going, as long as we were together, everything would turn out okay. That also has proven true.

One Less "Person" in the Body of Christ

Our departure to the West was unfortunately met with resistance from our local church leaders. For some reason, it wasn't in *their plans* for us to move. Interestingly, it was always in our plans. What happened in our process to conclude our lives in Grand Rapids, Michigan, went from *holy* to *woefully not so cool*. Somehow, the church leadership felt we were being selfish and simply wanting to do things our way.

That had a familiar felt sense of what I had experienced while being a member of the campus ministry group before medical school, and my experience when I was making my decision about medical school. I recalled how the church leadership treated me then. Now, while it was a different church, it still was the "body of Christ." Honestly, I was not up for that again. Knowing that I trusted Andy and the felt sense that I had about our life together, we respectfully stood our ground.

Suffice it to say, we were treated with much less respect than what we deserved and we were accused of "breaking covenant." I am not exactly sure what that means, but I do know how it felt to be told that. It was awful, belittling, and humiliating. In our departure from Michigan and re-establishment in Colorado, we made another monumental decision: We decided to discontinue our church attendance.

In fact, for me, that led to an eight-year length of time where I effectively threw the baby *and* the bathwater out (of the window), battened up the windows, and torched the house. I was pretty determined to never be treated in the same manner as that time and the times before. Anything that led to the felt sense of not being enough or doing enough in God's eyes, I wholly rejected. That was a long season. And I was pretty resolute in my reason for that season. I no longer wanted to not be enough for God. It would take some time, but that part did get sorted out, and I have found my faith again, but not in the same manner as before.

Life Lessons

Wherever you go, there you are. You are always where you are meant to be, because there you are. If you were meant to be somewhere else, you would be. So be patient with yourself, compassionate and understanding. Know that it is okay to struggle with your beliefs and faith. In the end, it will be all good. And if it is not all good, it is not the end.

Words to live by.

Chapter 5
Bone-Setters, Blow Jobs, and Hallowed Bones

"You've done pretty good for a girl of average intelligence."
—High school counselor, male

Concussions and TBI, not TMI

In high school, I did well, but I was a talker. I spoke out of turn and frequently talked to my classmates. Sometimes it was difficult to stay on task. Other times, because of great interest in something, I was hyper-focused. Nowadays, we call that ADHD. Back then, it was called being disruptive or not focused.

Then there was that concussion.

While riding my bike home from my friend Mary's house, I put my foot in the front tire spokes of my ten-speed bike. Not intentionally, mind you. My quick-release hub was loose and, like many times before, I tapped it with my foot while moving at a high rate of speed. That time, however, my foot went into the spokes and then the wheel rolled on. When my foot jammed in the spokes and the fork, I went flying over the handlebars and was knocked unconscious. Friends tell me I bounced on the pavement like a rag doll. I don't recall anything.

A very kind man pulled me out of the road and propped me up against a telephone pole. Amazingly, my neck was not broken, but I was rendered unconscious. When I came to, I remembered my name, phone number and address, and my dad's name. All of which I kept repeating, because I had retrograde amnesia—that means I didn't recall what happened to me just before my injury, or anything about the injury, for that matter. So I kept asking, "What happened?"

My parents arrived quite quickly, and right after them came the ambulance. It was Bud's ambulance, the best of the two ambulance services in our city. My dad rode in the ambulance with me and Mom followed in our car. I went in and out of consciousness, and still I kept asking my dad, "What happened?" He would tell me, and then a short time later, I would ask the same question again. My brain-injury version of wash, rinse, repeat. All told, I had a second-degree concussion, broken left clavicle, and a number of bumps and bruises. Everything healed well, except not really my brain, though I did not know that at the time.

For my upcoming year in high school, I enrolled in geometry. After that would be calculus. Additionally, there were chemistry and physics. But I began to struggle in school. Geometry was impossible for me. In class, it all made sense, but when trying to do homework or take a test, I struggled. I did okay with chemistry, as it was memorization. I didn't give calculus a go, because I got a D grade in geometry. There were consequences to my low grade: disappointment and not making the honor roll. I did not have headaches (miraculously) and my broken bone healed well, so that was more of a hidden residual of the bike accident.

I had some ups and downs in undergrad too, mainly with

math and spatial orientation. What I knew to be true was that in tenth grade, I did well on the standardized test for spatial orientation, but not on any subsequent test. And there was that less than stellar grade in geometry. Teachers thought I was just not focused enough, and that was true, but the concussion was not taken into consideration. It would be many years before I understood what had happened to my brain.

Medical School—My Calling

In the meantime, I pursued my goals, completed undergraduate and then some graduate school, and entered medical school. I was in heaven and wanted to be an orthopedic surgeon. It was then that I visited my high school for an alumni event and I ran across my high school counselor. That was when he proclaimed that I had done pretty well for a girl of average intelligence. At some point later, I met for lunch with a former high school teacher who was also my track coach. During high school, she was a mentor for me. We talked about the conversation and comment that my former high school counselor made and, since then, to this day, when she and I meet for lunch once a year, we both roll our eyes at what that counselor said.

In medical training, I loved the idea of fixing things, wearing scrubs, smelling of antiseptic, and putting on casts. Did I mention scrubs? I loved them.

In medical school, we spent a little over two years in the classroom, mixed with lab classes, and worked with preceptors in physician offices in the communities that surrounded our campus. Then we went to our base hospital for the remainder of our medical school experience. That meant our medical school class was scattered all over the state of

Michigan in various training hospitals. At the time, there were a significant number of osteopathic hospitals. Since then, many have merged with allopathic hospitals or closed. Even now, the residency training programs are combined under one umbrella for both MDs and DOs. Everything is consolidated. Medicine and the training for it is nearly unrecognizable now compared to when I was trained. I am sure that is also true on many other levels regarding medicine as well, but I digress.

At the time, medical school and our clerkships had a lot of key features, traditions, and characteristics that made us something of a tribe or a club. It was hard to gain admittance to that club, and I knew the high sign. I was in and belonged. What a feeling. It was that same felt-sense feeling, the one that resonated in my bones. I knew I was where I was meant to be.

Scut Monkeys and First Assists

Training as a medical student had a lot of unique aspects to it, and even more characteristics, depending upon which base hospital we were assigned to. The location, demographics, and specialties offered, in addition to the known attending physician, were all considered when making a choice of a base hospital experience.

I was assigned to a small town in the lower Upper Peninsula of Michigan. The number of residents there were two, then there were three interns, and three of us medical students. So the entirety of the house staff was eight. In other base hospitals in Michigan, there were five times as many house staff. Why that is important is because the more house staff, the more the hierarchy of the medical system plays a role. Medical students are at the bottom. We were called *the scut monkeys*. The term comes from the infamous book, *The House of God*, written by Samuel Shem. That book was then turned into the TV show *St. Elsewhere.* And it is all true, just as written.

Bone-Setters

I loved all of my training. Some days I felt confident, and some days were just scary, as I was doing things I had never done before, i.e., stitches, placing IV lines, inserting medical instruments into orifices, etc. Always learning, growing, and living in wonder regarding my profession. This is what I was born to do. And fixing bones felt that way too.

Because the house staff was limited, I had the very good fortune of being "first assist" on most procedures and for care of the patients. That meant I was very hands-on and worked right next to the training physicians, also known as attending physicians. They would be responsible for guiding and grading me for the rotations and specialties that changed monthly.

There were required rotations and electives. I filled all of my electives with orthopedics, aka *ortho.* Daily tasks were completed and then we were on our own for a few hours each day. Our schedule was 7 a.m. to 7 pm. Twelve hours, five days a week, and then every other weekend. Sixty hours a week and then give or take another twenty-four hours if the weekend call was needed.

What sorted out was that I was good at quick decision-making, judgment, and hand-eye coordination. That meant surgery. I loved ortho because, well, I just loved it. Standing at the sink in my scrubs outside of the OR, cap on, face mask on, and washing up to my elbows for five minutes was my kind of heaven. I loved the soap, the smell of the soap, and being clean. I loved the lighting, the usually blue tile walls, and the hushed reverence of putting the patient to sleep and then applying the sterile drapes just so over them so as to expose the necessary areas without the rest of the body being exposed. Definitely, there at that step is where the depersonalization occurs. I shall reframe that as compartmentalization, because getting singularly focused allows the surgeon to provide the known repetitive motions from hours of muscle memory as they execute the needed surgical technique. Yes, on a person, but, moreover, yes, in a systematic process.

Anatomy is known by location, location, location. You would think it was real estate, and in a way it kinda is. You move down the bone and the name for the section of the bone changes. When you describe this using medical terminology, you know exactly where you are. Left, right, medial, lateral, superior, inferior, tubercule, epiphysis, diaphysis, etc.

The surgical procedures are all well thought out and planned. Literally every move, retractor and instrument placement, cut, and/or suture is planned. Sometimes it is even timed. Surgery requires a symphony of movements by a number of team members with the surgeon being the "captain of the ship." What's not to love about that? As a medical student, I could not find any downside to it at all.

Because I was so focused on ortho, I spent all of my extra hours, weekend call, and rotations studying bones, fractures, the setting of fractures, and the naming of fractures, which is a whole lexicon in itself. In fact, there is a classic book named *The Language of Fractures*, by Robert Jordan Schultz. It teaches you how to name the fracture of a bone, or bones, based upon identification of the said bone, then the location on the bone of the fracture, then the type of fracture, then the characteristics of the type of fracture. Some fractures are named after the physician who identified the fracture, and some are named after the mechanism that caused the fracture.

It is all wonderfully complex, and when you understand the language, you are "in" the ortho club.

The attending physicians watched with great enthusiasm as my skills grew. They also appreciated that I gave attention to detail in the pre- and post-operative state of care, and thus they had a good worker under their tutelage. It was a win-win.

Working that hard provided a rare opportunity for me to complete a solo surgery as a medical student. That meant I was the lead surgeon, and the attending physicians were in the supporting role. As they were right there beside me, they could quiz, check, and double-check my every move and decision. I memorized the technique for the surgery, and I had to describe it in detail before I was allowed to take the lead. I was quizzed on what I would do if things went wrong—which, of course, they did not, but as always, a surgeon must be prepared. As the surgeon, I was going to perform a below-the-knee amputation. The unfortunate patient was losing his leg due to both diabetic and vascular complications. Prior to the operation, I spent time with the patient explaining the surgery and the post-operative care, and then carefully answered all of his questions.

When the surgery came, I was ready. The three of us physicians—actually, two physicians and one medical student—came together and completed a successful case as I systematically described the anatomy, the next required step, be it a cut, saw, or tie-off, cauterized, or sutured. In a good amount of time and without any complications, we were able to accomplish the amputation. It was not lost on me what type of surgery I was performing—I held a compassionate reverence for the simultaneous loss of limb and the saving of the patient's life.

Referencing the Reference Letter

After that, there were more bone-setting opportunities and there was more fracture-naming, and all along the way, quizzes and questions from the attendings. All the feedback was stellar, beyond good. "Well dedicated and conscientious" were the words I heard. "Beyond the level of her schooling." "She will be a great surgeon." I was in heaven. I was anticipating an excellent grade and, more importantly, an excellent reference for application to an orthopedic residency program.

I had a meeting with those surgeons to request the necessary reference letters needed for residency. The atmosphere felt uneasy. It was less open, and less friendly. They both asked why I thought I should become an orthopedic surgeon. Whereas I thought that was quite obvious, it apparently was not. I couldn't figure out why that type of conversation was occurring. However, what I was beginning to hear and what was being implied was that I should have done more "favors" for the attending surgeons.

These weren't direct requests by the attending surgeons, but rather vague suggestions of what could be provided by me in order to receive an excellent recommendation. Honestly, it was lost on me, what was being asked for, until there were more hints. And then I caught on that the favors were for things that were not related to medicine.

An attending physician's car could use a cleaning. That was framed with me doing more weekend work in the hospital, and then something quite unexpected in addition to those extra tasks that were focused on their personal needs. And that was a shocking one: a blow job. Yup, you read that correctly. A blow job for a reference letter. He seemed to sneak that in between the weekend rounds and car washes.

I was shocked, dismayed, and appalled. It *never* crossed

my mind that sexual favors were needed to get into residency or even just to apply to a residency program. Because we were casually sitting in the men's locker room between cases at the time, I first attributed the comment to the location—you know, locker-room talk. But then I realized he wasn't kidding. My face turned red and I stammered and looked at the ground. I quickly excused myself and waited by the scrub sinks for the next case to begin.

I never mentioned it again. When the time came for recommendation letters to be written, I received just an okay evaluation, not at all the same feedback I was initially expecting. How naive was I? Turns out, quite naive, because I went back to the attending and inquired as to the reason for the less-than-stellar reference. I was told that I should not think too highly of myself, as I still had so much to learn. *Ugh!* Seared in my memory is the event of the attending pointing to his anatomy (not orthopedic, but still referencing a bone) and me just wanting to shrink until I disappeared.

What was challenging to recover from (besides the obvious) was that since I had spent all of my time in the ortho world at that one hospital, I had no recourse. I had no other attending in my corner or any other orthopedic surgeon who knew of my skill and passion for ortho. Reference letters, phone calls, and physician lounge talk were equally as important as, sometimes more important than, our overall performance, especially if we wanted a highly sought-after residency position. It turned out I was naïve.

Hallowed Bones

After completing my base hospital requirements, I had the good fortune of being encouraged to study abroad for a few months. A mentor, Philip E. Greenman, DO, who literally wrote the book on osteopathic treatment (*Principles of Manual Medicine*) had encouraged me to consider a stint in Europe with some of his colleagues. Dr. Greenman knew I was deliberating between orthopedics and a non-surgical approach to orthopedics, osteopathic manipulation. Not wanting to manipulate me, he thought a broader exposure would be good for my learning. Little did I know that it would also be good for my soul!

Arriving in Zurich, Switzerland, just into the new year 1993, I was to stay with a family who lived about thirty minutes outside of the city. I was to work at Schulthess Klinik, a world-renowned orthopedics and neurologic hospital. Travel to the Klinik was by train, but I stayed in a farmhouse and each morning walked through the cow pasture to catch the train and did the same when returning home each day. The contrasts in environments was key to my experience. From high-tech hustle-bustle to the quiet Swiss countryside. It was lovely.

Because I did not know German or, in that location, Swiss German, I was a bit isolated during the surgeries. The usual operating room banter was absent. However, that allowed me to focus on the work and the steps of the surgery. There was no language barrier with naming of the bones and the instruments for surgery, nor was there anything lost in translation in the surgical process. It was the same process I had learned and excelled at in America. The Swiss surgeons appreciated my skill, and they had many compliments and words of encouragement for my stage of training.

Stepping into the Neurology and Rheumatology department and applying osteopathic treatment (European style) was also affirming and, again, I excelled in those areas as well. A bit more of a language issue arose, as the patients were awake, unlike surgeries where they were asleep. The education was a bit harder to obtain because of the language barrier, but I was able to sort that out.

Returning each night to the country farmhouse included a train stop in the village. There, I would hop off the train, pop into the small grocery store and buy my dinner and the next day's breakfast (bread, cheese, coffee, salad, meats, and more bread) and then catch the very next train to my needed stop at the farmhouse. It took an easy ten minutes to shop and catch the next train. I literally felt like I was in heaven. There was no driving, just an amazing train ride, where I watched the scenery go by, and a brisk walk in Zurich to the Klinik, then the same on the way home. That routine was helpful, because everything else was foreign, literally.

Most evenings in the farmhouse, I would read and prepare for the next day's schedule. I also flipped through the TV stations and found the BBC. It was the only English channel. All of other channels were in French, Italian, or German. Switzerland is unique with its languages, as they speak four languages, depending upon the region of the rather smallish country. Also, the German dialect was interesting, not High German, but Swiss German that was a bit more sing-songy.

Those circumstances created a bubble for me to exist in. Perhaps another view would be an isolation, as I was culturally, linguistically, and locationally isolated. I spent a lot of time alone, but I was not lonely. I had brought a few books to read. One in particular was titled *Practicing the Presence of God*, by Brother Andrew. It was a small paperback book about an ancient monk who spent a lot of time in silence before God. I guess that was why it was a small book. "Not much to say here folks. Move along."

That book was a Godsend. I read, re-read, and simply sat quietly for extended lengths of time. During that time of studying bones abroad, as it were, I felt the time was sacred and set apart. I had time to sit, listen, and simply be, after months, years, of a tremendous workload and learning schedule. Listening to my soul, to Spirit, I learned that I did not want to be an orthopedic surgeon, I wanted to work in a more general setting where I could use my skills to hopefully prevent a surgery. I desired my patients to be awake and not asleep, and I wanted a lengthier doctor-patient relationship, rather than a quick fix and then be done with the case/patient.

All of those requirements pointed away from a surgical specialty and to a more primary-care setting. Sitting quietly in the upper room of the Swiss country farmhouse, my calling, destiny, and direction felt sure. I had a strong felt sense of the direction for my career. No noise, no expectation, just the whispers of the soul and Spirit. It was settled.

The time in Europe has always held a special place in my heart for my experiences there. It was where, probably for the first time as an adult, I could sit quietly in Spirit's presence and not want to run away. Not want to hide nor feel ashamed. I simply was, and I simply experienced Presence, Love, Acceptance, and Belonging. And it was separate from my doing of anything. I simply was present. I simply was accepted. I simply belonged. I learned that I never was separate from God's love, it was only my perception that informed me of that. There was nowhere I could go that God's love wasn't already there. I was both surrounded by and enveloped in God's love and presence. It was a matter of a shift in perspective. A shift from fear to love. That, my friends, is a miracle, and as Brother Andrew called it, "practicing the Presence." It is a good thing.

My Soul's Lesson

I learned that I was not what I was to *do*. I was who I was called to *be*. I learned that quiet and stillness are a great gift and a beautiful way to live. I learned that no matter where I was, I was never without God. Ever. Never. Even if I felt isolated and foreign in a situation or circumstance, I could find, feel, and experience a felt sense of presence and peace that came from inside of me. I did not need the external stimuli or people telling me what I needed to do or who to be. I could daily do good work, learn, grow, and gain knowledge, and return to the quiet of my soul to connect deeply to myself and my source for answers to all of my questions. No interpreter was required.

Activity did not define me, but presence did. Being present with myself. Those months in Switzerland sank into my bones, and thus I gained hallowed bones in knowing my place and knowing myself. And it was so.

Chapter 6
The Javalina

"A yawn is just a silent scream for coffee."
—Author unknown

A Decade of Coffee

"Coffee, black, please. Yes, I would like a refill. Thank you."

That was my typical request from age seventeen onward. Coffee drinking was important to me in my senior year of high school, especially with early Saturday morning work hours. Not so much during the week, mind you, but on the weekends. Then, in Montana, when my parents owned the Sheridan Bakery, I drank coffee every morning because it was "time to get up and make the donuts." Coffee seemed necessary, and I liked the flavor.

In college, I used Folgers crystals and hot water in my dorm room. I had a small coffee maker that sat on top of my desk shelf. Truly, that was the best part of waking up. And I liked the flavor.

The University Center had great coffee too, and refills

were free! There, I mixed my coffee with chocolate milk for what was an early version of a mocha. I don't think we called it that, however. But I liked the flavor.

In the fall of 1983, I was in my professional program of athletic training and my study partner was Jill. At her house, we drank coffee that was even better—flavored coffees and real cream (raw milk) from a dairy cow. We had cinnamon, chocolate mint, hazelnut, chocolate cherry, etc. Lots of different flavors. I liked them all.

Those were the IWOG years. IWOG stands for Incredible Women of God. Or at least we thought as much! Our clutch of young women would meet, have a Bible study, do crafts (ahem, not me) and drink coffee. Lots of coffee. Move over, Folgers, the real stuff is here. And the flavors were great!

One spring break, a group of us drove from Missoula, Montana, to Seattle. Of course we visited Pike Street Market. It was there that I found my Nirvana: Starbucks! Lattes, cappuccinos, dark rich coffee (with no flavors). I was done with flavors and just wanted the "real deal." French roast coffee with cream. That was my favorite!

Mind you, all that time, I was not addicted to coffee, I just liked the flavor. Ahem. No follow up questions taken. Move along here, nothing to see....

Graduate school led me further into my love of coffee. That was the time when cafés and espresso began to take shape and spread out from Seattle to other regions of the country.

In medical school, I used to ride my bike to class and stop at the local café. I would grab a tall, double-shot, skinny latte and balance it on my handle bars all the way to my eight o'clock class. It was always worth the risky acrobatics.

Internship and residency requirements included coffee.

The shifts were long and there was a lot of work to do. Coffee was good and it made sense.

Visiting Seattle as a medical intern, I fell in love with all of the drive-thru coffee stands. What a brilliant idea. A lot of the different drive-thrus had their own brews and blends of coffee beans as well. It became clear how coffee beans were a lot like wine: from various regions of the world, with different soils, climates, and altitudes affecting the flavors and characteristics of the coffee beans. Then there were the types of coffee beans, either robusta or arabica. I was firmly in the arabica camp, typically a single-origin, perhaps a blend, primarily African, some Indonesian, but not so much Central American. Hmm. I had a palate for coffee—who knew?! What fun. I became passionate about coffee. I learned of its history, its medicinal qualities—ahem. Again, not an addiction, I just love the flavor, and I was a doctor by then, so always keen about the medicinal side of things.

And then I wondered... what if?!

Le Caffe Company—Following My Passion

What if?! What if I opened a drive-thru coffee shop? There weren't any around in West Michigan. It was 1994 and all things drive-thru were making their way, but not yet in West Michigan.

During residency, I was able to moonlight at the local urgent care facilities. I had a cash flow, had built a nice house, and was focused on graduating and getting a full-time job in Grand Rapids, and I wanted to start a business. I had the entrepreneurial itch. And I had a passion for coffee. So I researched out the idea of a drive-thru coffee stand.

Zoning and construction were two significant speed bumps in our township regarding location and structure for my business. But a mobile unit, like a trailer, had wide-open zoning possibilities and it was already constructed. Researching further, I learned of a company on the east side of Michigan that built something called the Javalina. It looked a lot like a wide horse trailer that was enclosed and it had a counter for walk-up service and a side for drive-thru or drive-up service. Hmm, what if?!

Cart (Javalina) Before the Horse

So I bought a Javalina, an espresso machine or two, beans, syrup, cups, lids, shirts, hats, aprons, business cards, and I was in business. Following Michigan guidelines and county health codes, Le Caffe Company was born in 1995. We launched in a snowstorm, on December 2, 1995.

Location, location, location. I had a great location: on a major inroad from the northern suburb into Grand Rapids, and the drive thru was on the right side, literally, of the road. The second morning a local merchant pulled up in the wee opening hours and raised Cain that we were in "his" parking lot. Not true. He was a tenant like me and we both were renting our space from the same landlord. The landlord made that abundantly clear to the other tenants of the strip mall and so I simply reinforced that concept. Especially when he asked me for the owner's information and I told him that he was speaking to the owner. He said, "*No way*. No woman could pull off something like this!" Ha. He obviously did not know who he was talking to!

Because I was mobile, with the Javalina literally on wheels, I was able to bypass the township zoning issues. Understanding that was a key component to the establishment of my business, and the landlords were fully complicit. We were all geeked to usher in the first espresso drive-thru in

West Michigan. Yep, you heard that right. Le Caffe Company was the first of its kind in West Michigan, and I started the business while I was in residency. What was I thinking?

Sidebar: Yes, a lot of people were wagging their heads at me, wondering why I wasn't content just being a physician. Didn't I have enough to do? But it wasn't about any of that. What I saw was that I had a passion, a vision, and... did I mention a passion? I was following my heart, fully. And people showed up to buy coffee, to work with me and for me, to expand our little enterprise.

Getting ready to open the shop, I realized that there was a need for a "Steady Eddy." The landlords knew of a guy who had recently moved to Grand Rapids to get into the coffee business, but was not working in the coffee business just yet. After a brief meeting, I hired Scott, who was from the Seattle area. His sister lived in Grand Rapids, so that was his connection from Seattle to Grand Rapids. Scott, or Scottie, as we came to know him, worked for me for a number of months. He was a great addition to the team, as he was a farmer who liked the early morning hours and was absolutely reliable: Monday through Friday. Boom (mic drop). Filling in the afternoon hours was done with high school students and some adult part-timers. It was fun, a lot of fun. A lot of work, a lot of learning, and a lot of fun.

We had our signature beans too! Through a local coffee roaster, I developed Le Caffe Company Blend. It was wonderful. The beans came from my favorite world regions, and they were the arabica beans grown at mid-altitude, roasted medium dark. Yum!

Just a note on our first employee, Scott. He became a friend of the family, then later dated and then married my sister. So, truly a good hire.

The Township Meeting(s)

So, the township did catch up to us. Remember, we were on wheels, so we were supposed to be clear of zoning issues. However, that was not how they saw it. Their lens was the tax and permitting lens: money. I was required to present my business to the township board for permitting, even though it was contrary to the township rules.

At the first meeting, my proposal was flatly rejected. They wanted the Javalina and Le Caffe Company out! There was no reasoning with them. I just got a flat rejection. I was fuming because they were flat wrong. Their objections were (ready for this?) that I was a woman, a doctor, and it had never been done before. From my perspective, none of that mattered, they did not interpret the zoning regulations correctly, and I was on private property. I had the protection of the landlord.

The landlord requested a second presentation for the next month. They coached me on how to present and what to present at the next meeting.

So, the following month, I showed up to the township meeting with diagrams and parking lot dimensions, knowing the zoning rules. My neighbor Ellen and the landlord went with me for moral support. I was nervous because, by then, we were a going enterprise, I had employed people, and there wasn't a better place on the north end to move the Javalina to. Plus, we had every right, and all permissions, to be located in the parking lot. The township's response and stance did not make sense. They were just being "the township," as their reputation had preceded them. The old boys club was fully functioning, and I was clearly not what they wanted.

Understanding what they had said the month before, I used those same objections to justify my position. *I was a woman*, so the township should support women-owned businesses. *I was a physician*, so I had a good position in the community. *It hadn't been done before*, and so far the concept was a hit.

One of the longstanding township trustees came to the second meeting. She was a stalwart in our community, and a family friend. I had not anticipated that. I had not even considered that. Being naive about how those boards functioned, I did not know that trustees held significant sway over the township board. I did not know what to expect.

When it came time for my presentation, I took a deep breath and gave my best pitch, as if the life of my company depended on it. Well, it did. After the presentation, the board began their discussion and raised objections again.

Then the trustee interrupted the discussion. She explained that she had known me personally since I was five years old and watched me grow up, that the township should, for all the right reasons, be proud and glad to have such a person wanting to conduct business in the township. She said their objections were unfounded and all permissions and permitting should be granted. Full stop.

You could have heard a pin drop in the meeting. It was silent until my friend Ellen began to clap slowly and then more vigorously and loudly, all by herself. She also let out a whoop and a woot! I stared at the ground in front of me. I was nervous!

With the trustee's influence, it was then settled. Le Caffe Company had all rights, privileges, and permits to be temporarily permanent at our present location. The caveat was that if I wanted another location (because I was on wheels), I had to get permission from the township before I opened my doors, or windows, as it were. Okay. No problem. Bye, Felicia! Off we went before anyone could further object.

We celebrated a great win, thanks to the support of our township trustee. Looking back, I seriously doubt my diagrams had anything to do with it! Rather, I feel that the truth prevailed, on all accounts.

Batter Up

One customer came along in mid-winter, just after we were getting established. He was the general manager of the minor league baseball team and asked us to come to the ballpark for the summer. Opening day was in April and we had only been open ourselves from the previous December. In five short months, we were considering expansion. So, we did.

In the summer of 1996, at the Grand Rapids White Caps ballpark, we had a coffee cart. That was a wild experience. You have about three hours to make as much coffee and as many lattes as possible in that time frame, seventh inning stretch included. I developed a White Cap-themed menu for the venue. We blended our syrups to make the beverages and named them The White Cap (a white chocolate cappuccino), Babe Ruth (a chocolate and caramel latte), Pinch Hitter (a cup of drip coffee with a shot of espresso), and The Mound (a combination of chocolate and coconut). They were very good lattes. We had a crew of five people per game to run the coffee stand. There were long lines, and it was a hit!

My mom particularly loved working for us, as that allowed her to have free entry to all the games. She proudly wore the company uniform, often brought her ball mitt, and chatted with all of the customers and other White Cap personnel. She was our brand ambassador. I paid her in beans, literally.

We sold a lot of lattes, and we employed a lot of people at a very fun venue all summer long. There was a lot of buzz about the venture and we had local TV coverage and stories, etc. Our team gained a lot of valuable experience working, problem-solving, setting up systems, and running things without me always being there. I was the vision, and they were the legs to the vision. A great combination.

At the conclusion of the summer, we declared the venture a success. Now let's define the parameters of that success.

Boxes checked in success column:

- Proof of concept
- Brand establishment and strengthening—more people found the Javalina
- Employment and training of staff
- Entertainment
- Community involvement

Profitability? Well, um, not so much. Because we needed so many staff members to produce the volume in the short time span of nine innings, including the seven-inning stretch, we netted $525.00 for the summer. My accountant and I chuckled as we reviewed the summer numbers together. Clearly, not a strong profit center, but our brand was strengthened, and we had made an impact in our community. Those were intangibles and priceless.

My Soul's Lessons

Not all profits directly impact the cash flow. The Javalina opportunity was a labor of love, and many lives were touched and changed. Young adults learned how to work, a concept was brought to life, and it spurred more coffee culture growth in our community. We created a stir with our unique approach to business, and I gained a brother-in-law.

Creating a business and running a business are two different things. They require a different set of skills and goals. The daily grind is great, but not my quadrant of brilliance. I am the visionary, positive disruptor, and risk-taker. Once the business is up and running, it is always good to have another person do the management and operations, as I will then be on to the next venture. I also learned to not apologize for that fact.

In the end, I hold the high honor of having the first drive-thru espresso stand in west Michigan—ever. We were the catalyst for the coffee culture to evolve in West Michigan and it was fun doing that. Starting and operating Le Caffe Company was a dream come true, and I am grateful for the experience and for that season in my life.

Chapter 7
Eating Cake with God—Finding Meaning When It Doesn't Make Sense

A dear friend of mine has twin boys. When she was twenty-four years old, she had a dream in which she saw two young men coming toward her during their high school graduation ceremony. They were her two sons who were graduating.

When my friend turned forty-two, she became pregnant and delivered twins: two boys. They are now growing up, and my friend has a lovely family.

My friend has asked her sons, "What took so you long to get here?"

They replied, "Well, we were eating cake with God." Seems reasonable.

My Story Is Different

Growing up, all I ever wanted to do was go to college, begin my career, and live a very happy life. While I was growing up, and certainly in early adulthood in college at the University of Montana, getting married was part of my plan, but having children felt ambiguous, as I wasn't sure I could sustain a marriage, given the home environment I grew up in.

My parents loved each other and they struggled. In the end, they were married thirty-one years, but most of those years were not happy. It was a difficult environment and caused a lot of doubt in my heart and soul regarding my ability to sustain a relationship. I did not have, nor was I taught, the communication or relational tools necessary. However, my parents did the best they could—that I know for sure.

Deep down in my soul, I wasn't sure I had it in me to be in a long-term relationship. My experience of my parents' marriage was of seasons in a unified family, followed by seasons of separation under one roof, with long droughts of limited and cold communication.

Thinking about having children felt even more ambiguous, for the same reasons, as there were seasons growing up when I did not feel wanted or accepted, especially by my mom. I learned later that was a result of her experiences as a child and the traumatic events that had made lasting impressions on her. Yet, I noticed the nagging ambiguity within my soul.

The eighties were wide open for women—well, wider open. There were a lot of changes with Title IX having occurred, and equality and inclusivity was expanding. I wanted a piece of that and wasn't sure how soon I wanted to "settle down."

In college at the University of Montana, I was keenly aware of the social structure and opportunities. As a young adult, I was involved in a religious community. I was, in fact, a "holy roller." More about that as we roll along, holy or not! In that religious community, I was taught that there were traditional roles of men and women, with the man being the head of the household and the woman being submissive. While that structure seemed more stable from what I grew up in, the thought of children made me very nervous. I wasn't sure I had the understanding, patience, and skill to raise a child.

Clearly, I did not want to repeat the patterns of my childhood, where I was not understood and at every turn it felt as if my intentions were questioned and held with suspicion. I was pushed to strict conformity from a young age. That did not fit my wild, imaginative nature. To be sure, as a child I never doubted my intentions or actions, which felt pure to me. I was happy being outside at every turn and in every season. I was alone a fair bit, but completely at home with my friends in nature, like trees, flowers, and rocks, and when playing basketball. My mom and others did not always see it that way. I was constantly asked, "You must be up to something. What are you up to?" I would reply in a cheeky manner with my height measurement and a hope for a few more inches. Harumph.

First Comes Love... Marriage... Baby Carriage

Andy and I met and married within a five-month span. That happened in my hometown of Grand Rapids, Michigan. We began dating in June, then were engaged in August, and married in November. It was after a few dates that our connection felt real, easy, and wonderful. On our wedding day, I had no doubts, fears, or anxiety. I was all in. Andy was too. Our relationship is now a quarter of a century old and it gets sweeter and deeper each year. Yes, there have been challenges—ups, downs, questions, fights, resolutions, and growth. Yet neither of us doubt our commitment and choices to this day. Andy and I met when he was thirty-two and I was thirty-seven. A lot of life had been lived separately, and when we met and fell in love, we thought that only good things were in store.

Each of us was established in our careers and life. Neither of us had been in a serious relationship for any length of time, as we had remained singularly focused on our careers. I had always believed that when I met the right person, I would know very soon in the relationship, and it would not be a long time from meeting to engagement and marriage. I figured, when you know you know. Ya know?

Andy and I thought that, most likely, babies would also come quickly in our relationship. We thought two kids might be a good idea, and it really did not matter if we had boys or girls. We just wanted healthy kiddos. In the initial stages of my marriage, I tried birth control pills, even the low-dose triphasic ones designed to mimic a menstrual cycle. However, they did not mesh with my body very well at all. I did not feel well while taking them, so after two months, they were discontinued.

On the Nest

It was about six months after getting married that I became pregnant for the first time. As a physician, yes, I knew the statistics of first pregnancies, age, and risks of miscarriages and was okay with what it meant clinically. While I did not anticipate anything but "all going well," I had professionally provided prenatal care and, therefore, I understood myself as a patient and had the cunning to connect with myself as an observing physician. I understood what I was facing as we began our early steps in the pregnancy and, while thirty-seven years old might be a bit older, it was not out of the question for pregnancy, as I had what was considered a negative gynecological history. Meaning, I had nothing that required treatment or care. All systems were a go. Or so I thought.

As the pregnancy progressed in the first trimester, my

apprehension about being a parent grew on the inside, seemingly at the same rate that the pregnancy grew. Daily, I felt an unease and sometimes a panic. *What was happening? What was going on?* I was not sure I felt up to the task, but the task was happening, and I needed to figure it out. Those were the same questions and issues I counseled patients through over and over as a physician. That was not news to me, but it felt like news to me, on the inside of my soul.

Perhaps, I reasoned, my ambiguity and apprehension grew because being pregnant was all new to me. As a physician, I had provided a lot of prenatal care and delivered many babies in my career. Mostly, that all seemed natural and miraculous, and yet, I wasn't sure about me birthing a baby and parenting a child. That was a strong, nagging feeling, a presence in my soul, and I could not discern where it was coming from. I did recognize it as the same doubts I had experienced when I yielded my locus of control to what others thought was best for me while I was in the various religious communities.

Ah ha, yes, there it was—it was the same feeling in my bones. No, it was in my soul, deep inside of me, or was I deep inside my soul. I wasn't sure exactly, but I had a *felt sense* that it was not right. I was doing something that I was monumentally unsure about.

My Body and Soul's Experience

What will my body do? What will I feel? What will my body return to after pregnancy? I kinda freaked out on the inside. While I had lost count of how many women I had comforted, counseled, and stood by as they progressed through the prenatal, natal, and antenatal periods in their pregnancies, and while I understood the science, OB/GYN guidelines, choices, risks, and various outcomes, I usually was witnessing a beautiful life entering our planet, joining the human race with all of the possibilities and adventures ahead of them. That was always an amazing journey to share with any patient. I learned early on that there clearly is both a science and an art to assisting a child to enter the world. And while all of that made a strong felt sense of the possible in me, I remained ambiguous and doubtful about my own pregnancy.

I carried the pregnancy for seven weeks and then I had a miscarriage. What I felt was sadness, fear, and relief. All at the same time. I remained curious about my relief and my ambiguity. Perhaps my body knew something. My soul certainly did. At the time, the relief did not consciously register, yet it was still a loss, a loss that we grieved.

Not Medicine's Finest Hour

Unfortunately, medicine by its practice is not kind to its own —physicians, especially—because while the miscarriage was happening, literally, I was on a shift in a local urgent care facility and could not leave to attend to my own acute needs. Irony is a part of medicine for all of us physicians. What we do every day butts up against our own life experiences. We care for dying individuals in one exam room and then in the next exam room counsel a woman on what to expect while they are expecting. I was having a significant medical event, the miscarriage was occurring while I was working in the local urgent care facility, and yet I could not attend to my own urgent medical needs, because I could not abandon my post. Irony.

Retrospectively, I realize that in that situation I needed to be taking care of myself, rather than taking care of others. I am sure there are laws about this, and I am sure that if I had acted to take care of myself things may have sorted out okay, but as it was, I started to pass the products of conception, my pregnancy, while working.

I was nauseated, dizzy, emotional, and crampy, all of which were normal and expected in the given circumstances. Having assisted many of my female patients in that situation before, I was aware of what was happening. As I sought relief from my employer, by asking to be removed from my shift and having someone finish the shift for me, I was met with resistance and push-back. Essentially, I was informed that I was to stay working, since they "couldn't find anybody" to cover the clinic. Basically, I was required to keep working. I was literally losing my pregnancy but was not allowed to go home and do it in a private setting with my husband. I was to stay put while I experienced a significant, life-altering event. I was told that if I left my shift, I would lose my job.

That event is important to understand, and I am sharing this part of my story to simply pull back the curtain on how physicians are treated differently from other patients. Who in their right fucking mind would ever tell a patient to stay working while having a miscarriage and not allow them to attend to their immediate needs?

Yet, in medicine, it happens all the time. Physicians must bear up under a lot of very strenuous circumstances and deny our own humanity in order to take care of others. We are restricted from going to the bathroom, eating, and sleeping, and must work long hours daily in a variety of circumstances that are all a part of our world. In my case, at that time, when I needed to be able to go home or to the emergency room, I was denied the opportunity to tend to myself. Not a good look for medicine caring for its own.

So I stayed at work and frequented the restroom. There, I privately cried, vomited, bled into the toilet, and lost my pregnancy. It was horrible. I had to get supplies from the urgent care for my bleeding. Meanwhile, patients were waiting. There was no relief in sight. At the end of my shift, I went home to Andy and collapsed. Together we grieved the loss of our pregnancy.

Looking back, I was afraid that if I walked out I would actually get fired. I don't know if that was true. It was what I was told, however. At the moment, in the trauma, I felt vulnerable on so many fronts, and I needed my job, so I stayed. The level of distress was extreme, but I also saw an end in sight—the end of the shift. It seemed that I was able to compartmentalize both my work and my grief, yet, overall, I was both miserable and grieving.

Questions of My Soul

During the short time of knowing I was pregnant, I noticed that I was able to experience a soul connection with the pregnancy. Interesting. Curious. But was that really what I felt? And, if so, how did that soul connection occur? Was it in the same manner that is known as a mother's love that is never-ending? Why was it so strong? Was it because I was only to know them for a short time? And why did the ambiguity play such a strong role? What did my soul know about my body and this pregnancy?

What I knew was that because of the loss of the pregnancy, I wouldn't see the life of our baby come to being on this planet. A part of me had died and a part of my husband had died when we lost our baby. It was a tremendous loss. We felt the loss. We grieved the potential that was thwarted.

Regarding the soul connection I experienced, I do not have any theology, definition, or science as to how or when a soul enters a person. I did not know, nor do I now claim to know, where that soul was at the time I was pregnant. Was the soul inside of me in the burgeoning pregnancy tissues? Hovering within the rapid cell divisions and brooding over the fetal development by way of embryology? Or was it outside of my body, around the room and simply awaiting term and the impending delivery to then slide into place somewhere quietly in our child's body. Maybe we are enveloped by our souls? Who knows? I claim that I hold no absolute knowledge of where or how this part of the mystery of life unfolds, regarding babies as they come into this world, or people as they are actually on this planet.

Yet my experience told me that I deeply held a felt sense of a soul experience with my pregnancy and anticipated child, which felt both very real and genuine.

The Shape of Grief

In that moment of loss, grief felt like a loss of opportunity. A loss of a possibility of what could be. It was not a loss of what *was*, as the pregnancy was not viable for a significant length of time. While, clearly, there was a loss and, clearly, there was an opportunity at life, it was for sure more of a possibility of what that life was to be.

Experiencing grief in that manner was very interesting. There weren't any milestones of that person or that soul, other than what I had connected with during that short period of time. I never felt a quickening, a jump, or rolling, but there was a lot of hope, and I had a soul connection and felt that there was a potential for life and a potential for the pregnancy to continue. But it did not.

Many people wished us well, sent cards, and provided condolences. Our families understood. That was kind. Until it wasn't.

What I learned was never to share with a woman or her husband after they've been through a miscarriage that, "Miscarriages happen all the time. The good news is that you have proven that you can get pregnant easily, so just try again." Those are inappropriate words of condolence. "Your child is in a better place. God needed them more than you did." *Yikes.* WTF? That does not make sense, nor is it an acceptable explanation. Even if miscarriages may be a common occurrence, there is still a significant loss. A grief that is real and felt and palpable.

What I know as a physician, as a person, is that the best response to a person's grief is to let it simply be witnessed. That's it. Each of our own relationships to grief is different, even between husbands and wives who experience a miscarriage. I promise, you don't even need to make additional comments. Just witness. Each life, each instance where grief occurs is unique. No circumstance or event is ever the exact experience of another person. Allow for space, time, and room for the emotions to occur, for reactions to develop within the grieving couple, and do not offer platitudes or words of wisdom to them. The power lies in the witnessing of the grief. People think that because they have had their own instance of grief that may seem similar, they have the right words, the answers, and the support that will make a difference. However, that does not automatically make it the same for anyone else. Each loss brings a unique characteristic arc and story. And the grief must be witnessed.

After the miscarriage, I was advised by my OB/GYN to wait about three months before attempting to conceive again. I trusted her as my physician because she was a colleague, a friend, and she specialized in high-risk pregnancies. Early on, she and I had decided that, no matter what, she was the physician for me because of our friendship and the bond that we shared as colleagues—not because I was high-risk or anything like that.

After the first miscarriage, my OB and I reviewed the events, discussed that often the first pregnancy is not viable for a variety of reasons, and that it would have been nice to have the aborted tissue so we could have done a complete lab analysis. When I shared my story with her of how my miscarriage unfolded, she was shocked that I had not been able to go home from my urgent care shift. She acknowledged how poorly physicians are treated when they become the patient. We also discussed that, indeed, I did conceive quickly. That was a helpful piece to the puzzle.

Work Will Help You Stay Focused—Band-Aids to the Wounds

During that time, I was being myself and thus starting another round of my entrepreneurial approach to medicine. I was opening a new private office. I had been wooed away from my clinic job into a different clinical start-up situation. It was a clinic that provided complementary care. They were backed by a number of private investors, and it was the first of its kind in our city. I was thrilled to be asked to be the medical director and lead physician. I was full of hope and very excited that I could learn more about integrative medicine and practice in a manner that really fit who I was and how I thought.

Unfortunately, the clinic struggled, and my posting was not what they had initially presented to me. Without any ill intention, the clinic as a start-up quickly lost all the money because the people in charge did not know how to run a medical clinic. What I know for sure is that a medical clinic is a unique beast in terms of how it runs, how to build it, and how to be successful. The margins are razor thin and it was a new idea for the community. So, while the idea was revolutionary at the time, the execution was horrible and, thus, that venture did not last. But I had left my previous employment position (yikes), except for the urgent care part, so I did what any entrepreneur would do: I hung out a shingle and continued to see patients and reinvent myself.

By that time in my career, I had really been impressed with a more holistic approach to medical care that cornered on the strength of the doctor-patient relationship. What that meant specifically was that I needed more time with patients, so my appointments became thirty to sixty minutes in length. Lengthening the appointments allowed me time to listen more deeply to my patients. I began to see how that was important because, in doing so, they *told me what was wrong with them.* What I was witnessing was my intuition and deep skills emerging and becoming a central part of how I practiced medicine.

A Felt Sense of Listening

Those skills and the listening were not limited to the exam room. My life was turning more and more in that direction. It became natural to hear, see, and understand at a deep soul level. Identifying with others' pain and experiences became the norm for me. I was blossoming into the empathic healer I had always thought I was.

With that experience came a feeling, a sensing of the three parts of me coalescing and acting as one: mind, body, and spirit. I would often consider the mind as the soul, not only the thinking part but the felt sense part that included thoughts and perceptions.

Stirring in me too were feelings that were slightly less ambiguous about children. After the first miscarriage, I realized that I had a lot of fears about being a mom, changes in my body, and what it would be like to be pregnant. What captured me the most, however, was the soul connection I had with our first pregnancy. That felt sense of connection was interesting, curious, and enlightening. The pregnancy felt very much feminine and a girl. She felt artistic, fiery, and sensitive at the same time. It was important to grieve that which I had perceived as my daughter, the felt sense of what could have been.

Next on the Nest

On the heels of that, I noticed that our next pregnancy felt like a little boy. Curly blond hair, bright blue eyes, and full—so very full—of life and exuberance. He felt like a natural athlete, intelligent, and with a deep sensitivity to life and those around him. I was eager to try to get pregnant again.

I wasn't pregnant when I felt those things and, well, it did not take long, because in the first month of trying, I was pregnant again. We did not announce anything. We wanted to wait until the first trimester was nearly completed before we let people know. My OB/GYN decided that we should do an early transvaginal ultrasound and check labs and other things sooner than later, because the first pregnancy ended in a miscarriage.

That proved to be a very wise choice, as my progesterone was very low. Progesterone is a female hormone that helps with the gestation and growth of the pregnancy in addition to the main pregnancy hormone, which is known as human chorionic gonadotropin. All other labs were great, so I just needed to take some prescribed progesterone to support the pregnancy. Seemed reasonable, and as the initial weeks progressed, I had the same sense of soul connection with the pregnancy that I had with the first pregnancy, although I had stronger feelings of it being a boy, with lots of perceptions of his likeness and beingness. The bonding was swift and deep on that one. Interesting.

During the first trimester, I noticed changes in my body. With the extra progesterone on board, I actually felt quite good. I had minimal nausea, and certainly no morning sickness. My sister and I had a scheduled trip abroad to attend a friend's wedding in the UK, and even with the travel I was okay. Not too tired. Some of the people we visited seemed to be able to sense that I was pregnant, yet I was pretty well mum about it. I wanted to hold the secret a bit longer to, perhaps, in a way, help ensure that all would go well.

Actually, I am not sure that my friends actually sensed anything. It was probably obvious because I was not drinking my usual gin and tonics and martinis that I was known for. I am not sure they could read too much into me having a pregnant glow or anything. I just told them I wasn't drinking because of the travel time.

Shortly after returning home from the UK trip, about a week or so later, I developed some cramping and spotting. It was during the day, and I was in my clinic seeing patients. When I rang up my OB/GYN, she said she felt that I should come directly to her office to be examined. I did, after I finished with patients. It was only a short length of time, perhaps an hour or so. Even though there were some abnormal signs, I really did not have any symptoms. I felt good. I was excited and full of hope. Andy met me there, just in case.

An ultrasound was completed in the office, and it was determined that we could not locate a heartbeat. I was nearly eleven weeks pregnant. Surely, there was a mistake. Surely, it wasn't happening again. Surely, I had really made a soul connection with my son and I wasn't going to have another loss.

In fact, what surely happened was that I had lost the pregnancy. My heart was broken. Andy's heart was broken. We simply held each other and wept.

Searching for Meaning

Questions abounded. How could a love so deep that Andy and I shared not create and sustain another life? Surely, we had enough love. If love was the key ingredient, ours was vast and deep and profound and passionate. *Why is my body doing this?* I felt a sense of betrayal from my body, and I felt too that perhaps I had betrayed our child, failed to protect her, even in the deepest part of me, during such a vulnerable time. That was me as a mom. As a physician, I thought I should know better. That was a curious thought, that somehow, as a physician, I was supposed to know more about the process. Yet, at the same time, I had sensed a deep level of betrayal. I did not speak of that betrayal for many years. I buried it deep in my body as a result of the traumatic loss.

When the fetal demise was identified, it was recommended that I have dilation and curettage (D&C) to remove the products of the pregnancy and to have tests run. Surely, there would be an explanation and then an understanding and then a treatment plan and... and... and.... My heart was very broken.

Suddenly, it became clear that my choice of physician, my friend and colleague, *was* the best choice for me, as it sorted out that I most likely was a high risk for pregnancy. The jokes we had made weren't funny anymore. My only thought before about being high-risk was that I was going to pretend to be high-maintenance and want to be waited on, pampered.

Then, later, instead, I did need comfort and consolation and compassion. I was the patient and not the physician who was typically in charge of situations. I had no control and I felt powerless, vulnerable, and scared.

It took about one month to get all the labs and analysis back. The tissues were sent to a lab on the East Coast that specialized in fetal demise and included genetic testing and a full pathology report. Certainly, we would get to the bottom of the problem.

The report showed that we were having a boy, just as I sensed. But what was odd was that there was not a single syndrome that emerged from the chromosomal pattern to provide an explanation regarding the why of losing my pregnancy. The report was inconclusive. The genetic pattern of the pregnancy was simply "incompatible with life." That meant: no fancy name for it, no understanding of why, and no next steps, because the pregnancy was simply incompatible, at odds with, out of step with, contradictory, ill-matched, unsuitable for use together with me, because of chemical interaction or antagonistic physiological effects. Incompatible.

Physician Understand Yourself

The labs result was very difficult. It cut deeply and to the quick of my soul. Moreover, as a physician, somehow, I felt that I was supposed to know better. Again, there was that thought. Curious. *This wasn't supposed to happen.* Okay, once perhaps, or even perhaps twice, especially around week five or six. But certainly not after week ten.

A mix of heartbreak, grief, guilt, and shame became my constant companions. The self-doubt took a deeper hold. My faith in God/religion was shaken. I did not enjoy the condolences of the "trusted others" who seemed to know so many right things for my life. I listened to my soul, and I wanted out. But I wasn't sure. I knew that I wanted out from under the watchful eyes and gazes of the trusted others.

Being a physician is quite powerful, from an ego standpoint but also from an empowering standpoint as well. Having answers, insight, and skills, and affecting outcomes were what I did best. My situation, however, was beyond me. It was out of my control, for sure.

There was a deep need for me to be a physician to myself in that setting, just as I used my gift and skill to help others. A lesson for the physician healer was simply this: *Physician, heal thyself. Listen to what I need, what my soul wants, and not what other people think.* Interestingly, that story goes back to my pre-teen years and continues pretty much throughout my entire life. It was continuing to be a theme in my life. From the many traumatic experiences and illnesses I had, I was learning to heal myself by listening to myself. I was reconnecting with my soul.

Later Lessons for My Soul

Upon reflection of those circumstances from a vantage point that was much later in life—twenty-two years later, in fact, I learned that I did not know exactly how to heal myself regarding the miscarriages. I needed help because of the trauma being held in my body. I could not see, and I did not know at what point or where I stepped off and abandoned my self-compassion and self-trust, exactly, but it seemed to be conjoined to a desire for connection and acceptance with others.

I learned that I still was concerned, some twenty-two years later, about what others thought about my choices and my desires, and not what my soul's journey was. As a youngster, I had a sense of being, of connection with myself and with nature. That connection felt surer when I was a youngster than it did after I experienced more life, conditioning, expectations, various illnesses, trauma, and loss.

As I grew, I unfortunately believed that belonging meant I needed to conform. Trust me, I would try time and time again to conform, to be a part of the group, clique, or clan, and then something would go horribly wrong and I would experience a significant disruption in my relationship and, thus, my life.

While I don't think the miscarriages were a mistake, I did begin to question my desire for a family. Thinking about being pregnant again as the possibility of a miscarriage was not something I wanted to sign up for. So, we paused. The ambiguity became a louder voice again, so pausing felt like a good idea. And it was.

I also was experiencing increased self-doubt about many things in life, and that had a firm hold upon my soul. The information and words, the insight that came from outside of me had seemed more valuable than my own internal guidance. My religion was saying that I couldn't trust myself, my body, and that God's plan was bigger, better; that I needed a bigger faith, a more committed heart. I needed to do more to get more from God.

My doubt was not only whether my body could carry a pregnancy, but also did I want to carry a pregnancy? That was a looming question—it was a soul question. One for the ages. What did I really feel by connecting deep within my soul? That part was difficult because of the traumatic event of the miscarriages and not fully healing or integrating my experience. So, accessing my true feelings was nigh impossible, as I was disconnected.

Now, many years later, being trauma-informed, or trauma-trained, I have come to understand that we cannot have connection to others without first being connected to ourselves. It is not possible. We are hardwired for love, belonging, and connection at a soul, spiritual, and body (soma) level. That is our natural, divine, organic state. Trauma disrupts that connection. It frays the wires between the soul, body, and spirit. The disconnect occurs because it is too painful to stay connected, so we dissociate. It is safer, easier, often lifesaving —and dysfunctional. Sometimes, that disconnect, with all of its tethering, is the only way we stay on the planet. We cannot reintegrate because the nervous system is blocked, our emotions are blunted or buried or cut off, and we are merely operating on autopilot and watching our life go by instead of living our life.

If we are not connected on the inside with these three areas, then we dissociate from ourselves. If we are not connected to ourselves, we cannot connect to others. We have a lot of neuroscience and behavioral science to explain this. I did not know this then. At that time, I knew I had failed, and I did not know why. The failure felt immense. How could a love so great not procreate? Andy and I had a profound love that was not reproducible. My body felt off, but then so did my spirit and soul. I certainly was not connected. Autopilot. Watching my life... go by.

After that loss, we decided to not try for another pregnancy too quickly. I was still grieving, and I did not want to fail again. Right? Wasn't that what was going on? Wasn't I having failed pregnancy after failed pregnancy? Why was a new life incompatible with my life? How was I at odds with myself and, moreover, *why* was I at odds with my pregnancy and perhaps even myself? Those were deep soul questions that caused me to re-evaluate my entire life and purpose.

The answers were not easy to come by. It took many years to understand the questions. A cloud was brewing, the cloud of the *unknown*, and it had a sprinkling of ambiguity along with it. That was beginning to be a familiar companion to my life's journey—my search for answers and meaning at every turn. Somewhere down the road....

Work, Baby, Work

Life otherwise began to move along, and I dug into my work again. My clinic in Grand Rapids was growing and I was approached to be "bought out" and join a larger clinic in our community. It seemed like a very good choice to do so, and so my shingle moved across town and my patients followed. I was digging deep into becoming an integrative physician and loving every minute of it. Andy was traveling for his work and so we simply put the idea of a baby on hold for "a while."

That "while" turned into months, then waiting for us to make a major move across the country for Andy's work, then waiting for us to get settled in a new community, and then waiting for us to get our feet under us with new jobs and opportunities. Suddenly, two plus years had gone by and we had not tried again for a baby. I simply kept putting off trying again. I could not face the idea of failing again, of incompatibility and all that went with the grief and loss we had experienced. And my faith was changing. I was changing. The ambiguity was back and I wasn't sure I wanted children after all.

Andy and I were long enough into our relationship that some dysfunctional communication patterns emerged. I freaked out. My parents had such a long on-again/off-again marriage that I was fearful of the same yet determined to not repeat their pattern. And continuing to wait on trying for children remained a constant.

For me, adoption was never an option, just not my cup of

tea. Hats off to all of the adoptive parents and families, but not what I was interested in. As for the dysfunctional communication, Andy and I headed to therapy. Imago therapy and understanding how to get the love we were seeking. It was transformative. Neither of us came from a strong family-communication background and many aspects of our communication had a dysfunctional pattern, so we had a lot of learning to do. Yet our love was deep and long and intense, so we simply did the work.

My Soul's Lessons

Therefore, as time continued to pass—weeks, months, one year, then two years plus—it became clear that my ambiguity for the idea of a baby was more than a passing thought; it was something I chose to listen to. As I contemplated my future, I was okay with not having children. Listening deep within my soul was accomplished by walking in nature, that time in the mountains. As I walked and connected with nature, I began to reconnect with myself again, in a deeper, more peaceful, and yet familiar sense. I was content with my marriage and career. I really loved my career, and I honestly enjoyed the freedoms we were having as a couple to come and go as we pleased. Being unencumbered was a lifestyle that seemed to suit us. I was able to remember the soul connection I experienced with the two pregnancies I briefly held. That proved to be a comfort, and my life would go on. It seemed right. It was okay. I was okay.

My outlook on life was changing too. I no longer felt beholden to what other people thought. Living in Colorado opened a lot of room for new ways to relate to myself and others. The struggle for my faith became real during the loss of our children, and it made me question many more things. It is safe to say that I entered both the dark night of the soul and the cloud of ambiguity in my beliefs. That phase would be a long and arduous journey and was not completed at that stage of my life. It was a relief that at least we were not raising children during that time frame. It was a huge relief, to be honest.

Passive Choices Worked

I came to understand that by not deciding about children, we actually had made a decision about children. We passively allowed time to go by, and the months and years helped mellow the hurt and provided space for us to find our feet as a couple who did not have children. We were okay with that. I was able to find peace in my soul knowing that it all worked out as it should.

The whys did not come immediately—it would take several years, but they did come, and there was even more in store for me regarding my soul encounters with my two children, but that's a story for another chapter.

In the meantime, I sat in the cloud of unknowing and ambiguity. It was an active sitting, mind you, with times of soul-searching, contemplation, and exploration of religious thoughts and dimensions. I opened to the idea that, no matter what, I was always and only ever going to be okay with God. I did not have to prove anything. In fact, honestly, regarding my religion, I threw the baby out with the bathwater, ran out of the house, torched the house, and flipped up both middle fingers regarding the whole idea of religion, especially all I had believed, was taught, and had experienced. I was now in the Wild West regarding my faith. It was wide open and ready to be explored... or not. It just did not matter anymore.

I began to understand that, no matter what, I *was* perfect, not flawed, and I only wanted exposure or thoughts of unconditional love about God. No performance, no promises, no kingdom mandate—and certainly no specific and fantastic plan for my life. Hell to the *no* on that one. Instead, I found that I was connecting more with nature again and with the stirrings of my soul that I recalled from my youth, even my early youth. Those experiences, those times of contemplation and practice of presence, helped me understand and heal, and to be okay with us being "empty nesters."

By reconnecting to my youthful soul experiences, I was able to sit quietly with spirit and accept more fully what had occurred with my body. The contemplation part of my journey continued for many years and became transformative to my career and approach to being a physician. The inner guidance became more constant in my work. However, in regard to church attendance and what I had known as religion, I was ruined.

Unlike my dear friend, whose story I told at the beginning of this chapter, I did not have the experience of knowing the dessert preferences of my children. I nonetheless experienced the essence of their souls and spirits. Ultimately, with time, curiosity, ambiguity, and a gently held trust, I was able to reckon with those truths and find peace in my soul, knowing that the two children were once a part of our lives and at the same time a part of the eternal world. To me, that seemed reasonable.

Chapter 8
Ceremony Number One

"The burning bowl ceremony is a fire ceremony that helps you release old, unwanted conditions or events in your life. Through the powerful and symbolic release of the burning bowl ritual, you can let go of anything holding you back."
—Google AI

On the morning of a full moon in Virgo, the snow moon, I arose early to seek clarity and solitude and soul work. I had left off the night before reading the book *Untamed*, by Glennon Doyle. She questioned what was perceived by herself and many others as a departure from God, Source, Herself, Spirit, Faith. As she reckoned with it, clarity came by way of understanding that she left *religion* and took God with her. God was not separate, nor was she separated from God. Essentially, she was protecting the truth of her Love roots and God roots inside of her that had been her Truth all along. What she was leaving behind was dogma, teaching, opinions, and trusted others who felt they had the answers for her life, as well as the answers for the collected others (other religious people). Because they were leaders, when they spoke, we listened, we believed. Until we didn't.

By using a ceremony, one has a way to bring an end to what needs to go, perhaps once and for all. For me, the first ceremony was years ago, and it had proven to be the first of many.

Prologue to Ceremony One (Circa 2002)

I was exhausted from it all. The politics, the games, the misinformation, and notions that in order to live well we needed to be full-on for God and believe in a very certain way. Holding a leadership position in the church and being seen as a leader was all well and good, until I was asked to do some things that were not in my integrity. I was asked to have the lead pastor step down and resign. I was on the deacons' board, but not an elder (primarily because I was a woman). Apparently, I was good at administrative leading, but not spiritual leading. In my heart, I wanted to serve, and so I did, in any capacity I felt I could and was inspired toward. But when it came to essentially firing a seasoned pastor, who, by the way, was married and had six kids and was the man who married Andy and me, I was not the gal for the job. When declining the task, I was asked about my commitment to the church and the Kingdom of God. *Whoa... what?* I did not see what one had to do with the other. It was subtle, but manipulative. Telling.

As that was unfolding, Andy and I were contemplating our next steps as a family. We had been married for a couple of years and 9/11 had just happened. We had the season of grief with the miscarriages, and we were on hold for a family. We knew that we needed to be in a city that was more tech-oriented and a place where, if Andy's jobs needed to be changed, we wouldn't be moving but rather he would only change employers. As a family medicine physician, I was kinda like a wedge: useful, and I could fit in anywhere. All points indicated to go west, to Colorado.

We made our plans and organized our next steps. In doing so, we felt open in our hearts, excitement, adventure, and anticipation. All good things. Yes, we would miss our family and friends, but the mountains were calling (again) and we must go. Our family and friends were excited for us and understood the necessity of the move due to Andy's work, and they were already planning visits.

We decided to move to Colorado and live in the Front Range area. We were going somewhere, just the two of us, and in many ways it felt like pioneering. We *were* pioneering, at least for our family and relationship. It was a sweet time.

As for the family visitors, true to their word, they visited. The first round was a mere five days after we moved in, and then my brother's family visited that summer. "We came in like a plague of locusts," my brother declared. It was all good.

But back to our departure. That was where the challenges really were.

Winding down my many physician responsibilities before moving took a lot of effort. Relocating as a physician involves getting licensed and credentialed and having background checks, and that all takes time, a lot of time, to accomplish. It is not just a quick check of a couple of references, or giving a two-week notice. No, the process is arduous and tedious. Typically, it can take 90 to 120 days, sometimes longer if there are malpractice issues to explain and such. My record was (and is) clean, so that was not an issue, but still, getting established in a new location is a thing.

The same was true for leaving the old location, as I had to extricate myself from insurances, hospital staff, committees, professorships, university teaching assignments, and board positions.

Then there was the local church. That turned out to be the more difficult part. The transfer of my professional life went off without a hitch. Not so much with the church.

Religious Responsibilities

I was on the deacons' board, an administration role, not a spiritual role. Because I was a female, it was okay for me to be on that board, as it did not carry any spiritual implications. My term would be up in the late summer, very near the time we were to move west to Colorado. Inevitably, continuing on for another term would be in order, but I felt comfortable and confident in our decision to relocate as a family, and so the completion of my board term also felt in line with my and Andy's decision-making.

What became interesting was that some of the elders (spiritual leaders) had begun to marginalize me due to my refusal to agree to a task that they wanted to give me as a member of the deacons' board, the task I mentioned earlier, to fire the current and longest-standing pastor. They reasoned (at least, they told me) that since I knew the man well, the task would be good coming from me.

Just before the decision to terminate the current pastor, they brought in a new pastor and, in making that decision, they subsequently concluded that they wanted to go beyond bringing in pastoral support and do a full replacement and redirection. I was unaware of those plans. The goal had changed from having the current pastor also remain on staff, to releasing him instead. It was sticky politically, spiritually, and ethically (the ethics were my issues).

Religious Structure

The larger church structure included elders, prophets, and apostles. They led from near and far, and were a strong and singular influence on the direction and growth of the church. As things were going, with being newly married and growing and changing myself as a result, that no longer resonated with me. I was not wired to be so charismatic and bombastic in my worship, and I couldn't see how I could continue to attend when more and more things seemed to go against my faith, which was built on loving God and loving your neighbor as you love yourself. I was struggling with loving myself after going through the miscarriages, and I was struggling with what I believed. It no longer felt in alignment with the Kingdom of God coming to earth as in a manner of dominion and lording over others with beliefs and doctrine. I was keener on loving and accepting and including, not excluding and judging.

As a result, Andy and I pulled back a bit in response to the changes at the local church. As we did, we felt more freedom in our hearts and believed that our move out to Colorado was inspired by our faith and beliefs. It resonated in all parts of our being—body, soul, and spirit. We were good with it. We were settled.

Andy recalls that we gave a lot of items away, many of them going to the new incoming pastor and his family. In doing so, Andy spent time with the new pastor. Because we had moved more to the periphery in our church attendance and responsibilities and we were getting ready to move, we spent a lot of our weekend time preparing and saying goodbye to our family and friends, so our attendance to the local church dropped off. However, Andy and the new pastor concluded that we would attend a particular Sunday service, and we would be blessed and sent out from the local congregation to our new home in Colorado. That was a ceremony. A closure, a change onward in a new direction. It was customary.

When the send-off ceremony Sunday came about, we set off for the morning service with a bit of nervousness and anxiety. We held out hope for a good send-off, even though I had refused to agree to the request that I fire the senior pastor, and I was not looked upon in a favorable way. My refusal stood on the grounds of integrity and ethics. What the elders wanted me to do was not part of the original discussion, strategy, and financial plans discussed when we were considering a new pastor. Then, after the arrival of the new pastor, firing the senior pastor had seemed to some of the elders like a *normal* next step. Retrospectively, me thinks that was the original intent all along, but I have no proof, only my intuition.

Because of the "hullabaloo" over that, I had resigned the positions I held and discontinued any leadership roles or tasks, as well as pulling away from basic attendance. That just happen to coincide with our decision to move to Colorado. While many people knew why we were moving, they were unaware of my stance on the issue of the senior pastor and how those events unfolded. Therefore, they were also unaware of why we seemingly stopped our overall participation as well. Coming back for the send-off, made sense and folks were eager to see it happen (in a good way—ahem).

As the regular church service unfolded and the time came to be "sent out," others had their time in the ceremony, but Andy and I did not. We weren't a part of any ceremony, as previously agreed upon.

The others who were making major life changes were called to the front of the congregation to be honored, blessed, given gifts, and prayed over. That was the ceremony part. That was the honoring of being a part of the church family. That was what Andy and the new pastor had agreed upon. Andy, in particular, felt that the church would want to do that, as I had been such an active member for so many years. He personally felt new still, but understood the friendships and relationships I was leaving, and he wanted to see it through.

What happened next was astounding. We were simply mentioned at the end of the ceremony part of the service: "Oh, yeah. Andy and Mary are moving too. This is their last day with us." That was it. That was our ceremony of being sent out.

Covenant-Breakers—Or So They Said

After the years of shared religious life together and being a part of a community, a church family, that simple mention at the end of the ceremony happened! The wind left me, as if from a gut-punch, and I could barely breathe. I wanted to scream, cry, run out of the building. But I froze. I just stood there as tears welled up in my eyes. The air was sucked out of the auditorium too, as a collective gasp and breath-holding occurred across the congregation. Yes, quiet as a church mouse, pin-dropping silent.

One of the elders/deacons whom I had long served with, stopped the service at that moment and requested to back up, giving a "Let's do this right" statement. That only made it even more awkward, and I lost more air from my lungs. Then, the gentleman who called for a stopping of the service stood up and led a prayer, and Andy and I were then seen as "sent out."

But what really was communicated through that service and then later through the grapevine (the Christian term for *gossip*) toward us and about us was that we were covenant-breakers. Covenant-breaking equaled breaking a vow, which by the way, we had not taken toward any church. Because we were leaving the community for work, that was seen as a selfish reason and showed that we were not following God. Again, me thinks that is more related to me taking a stand against the elders and my refusal to do their dirty work —the egregious firing of the (now former) senior pastor.

Baby and Bathwater

Following our relocation to Colorado, our experience of being away from that congregation was supportive of an "out of sight, out of mind" type of connection, or lack of connection.

The church people from Grand Rapids did not make any phone calls to us, ever. *Ever*. No visits, ever. Not even from the people I had been in contact with two to three times each week. They seemed to throw us out versus sending us out. Kinda in a baby and bathwater way. They were done with us completely.

During the initial year we were gone, a mere three months later, we did receive a few Christmas cards. But no phone calls. I did call people that I seemed to be close to, or thought I was close to. But they never called me, ever. I had to reckon with the one-sided pattern and make some choices. It felt as if we never existed. And I was hurt, deeply. I was devastated, broken, angry, and over it. I was done.

In Colorado, shortly after all of those events unfolded, I

made a choice to walk away from my religion. It felt so deep that I had a ceremony to commemorate the event.

As I stood in the yard of our new house in Colorado, I recognized my feelings—the hurt, betrayal, pain, and grief, and I was just over it all. I wrote down all of those feelings on paper, placed them in a pie plate, and struck a match. That ceremony was to rid me of my religion. And then I took some extra precautions (steps). I not only wanted away from all things related to God, I wanted to clear the decks, to start over, maybe, but just not yet. And, frankly, I did not know when. So the match was struck and the burning occurred. *Whoosh.* I released all things related to God (that I could think of). I wanted freedom, and to be left alone. Over and done with,

It felt like I threw the baby *and* the bathwater out, then I boarded up the house, torched it, and flipped both middle fingers up as I walked away. I was done. *Done* with church, church people, believing in God, and any kind of thing that smacked of religion. I was pissed off, big time.

I battened down the hatches to my heart about evangelicalism and church attendance and did not give one flying fuck about beliefs that I had held and faith that I held and the church that I had been a part of and... and... and.... I went on to live my life. For the next twenty-two years.

My Soul's Lessons

That ended up being a protracted season. I learned the lesson many years later, not necessarily at that moment of leaving the church and religion. At that moment, I was *out*, as in *Shark Tank* out. Not gonna believe. Full stop.

Instead, I opened my heart, mind, soul, and spirit to many views, belief systems, and experiences over the ensuing years.

I willingly listened and read and sat with different views than what I had previously held. And I learned to swear, a lot. That felt great. My mom did not particularly like it, but I did, so that was what mattered.

What I learned, what I got a felt sense about through the next years, was that my soul is eternal—no beginning, no end. Eternal life doesn't start when we die and leave this earth. It is eternal. It did not start when I came to this earth. It is eternal. When I got in touch with that concept and let it find a home in my body, in my soul, I quieted. What I was seeing emerge again was my trust in the felt sense of my body, soul, and spirit. It was contemplative, quiet, open, and connected to something much greater than myself that was both within and "without" myself, meaning outside of myself. And I felt at home with it, very much so.

Until then, I had held so much anxiety about my life and making sure that I found my life, didn't miss my life, made my life count, etc., that I had difficulty *living* my life. You might call it spiritual FOMO (fear of missing out). The anxiety was getting crippling. But when I returned to the felt sense of the eternal soul, I quieted. I was able to find and hold presence and Presence. I was connecting to something much bigger than myself and my worries. I was connected to Love, Source, Spirit, Universe. Then I could sense the connection to others as well. So, I sat in silence and quieted my soul. I became contemplative in nature. That meant that I also returned to the out of doors for quiet. Sitting by and under trees, along mountain streams, on big boulders, just being. Kinda like sitting in the lilacs when I was a kiddo.

I simply followed that for the next months and years. I gave myself permission to have no rules, other than following my integrity, which I had determined would come from my soul and trusting myself. Inherently, I possessed a strong moral compass of right and wrong, albeit somewhat judgy and self-righteous. So, I dropped that last part and let everybody and everything be as they were and as it was. That too felt really good, and really authentic. Then began my life again as a non-church-attending, non-evangelical, spiritual person.

From there, I learned a lot about ceremony and had many more ceremonies in the following years and decades that followed. I reckon I probably have done ceremonies throughout eternity.

Chapter 9
Swimming in Heaven—A Soul's Sovereignty

"To be sure of something is to have a conviction. To have an inkling is the same as your intuition. I had both."
—Mary Louder, DO

Mom's Story About "The Big One!"

I was jumping out of the car at the departure area of the Denver International Airport as my phone rang. It was 11:30 p.m. and I was getting ready to take my red-eye flight east to Maryland. I was to be at a conference in the a.m., attend for thirty-six hours, then fly to Florida to begin a five-day vacation with my husband and his sister, brother-in-law, and two nephews. We were going to Disney World. It was all planned and the details were sorted. I was looking forward to both medical education and then an epic vacation.

I could not discern if I had made a butt-dial or if my sister was calling me. It was 1:30 a.m. in her time zone and, as they say, nothing good happens after midnight. But mostly, she is always in bed early. Always. And she was calling me. It was not a butt dial.

It was the type of call that you never want to be on the receiving end of. Catastrophe. My mom was in the emergency room and she had suffered a trauma. At her bedside was my older brother and younger sister. Mom sustained a traumatic dissecting aortic aneurysm. The aneurysm began at the root of her aorta (where the artery originates at the heart) and extended down through her chest and into her abdomen, where it then divided into her hips, or iliac arteries, then into the beginnings of her femoral arteries, going into each leg. She called 911 herself and had been transported to the ER by ambulance, where they contacted my siblings.

This is the big one, a vascular trauma that approximately thirteen percent of the population survives. And it takes a village and a long time for the thirteen percent to survive.

Survival statistics of this type of vascular trauma is deciphered in an odd way, it is in days, months, and years, combined with many other factors. However, the farther out you go from the date of the trauma, the lower the survival rate. Overall, the odds are not good. And they go down with age and other factors that we physicians call *comorbidities*. Those are the concomitant diagnoses that people have, like hypertension, high cholesterol, inflammation, tobacco use, lifestyle issues, family history, etc. There is also a genetic component to an aortic aneurysm. Mom's older brother had a significant aortic aneurysm. We were unaware that Mom had any aortic issue. She was unaware of any aortic issues.

Her aortic injury was life-threatening, lethal if she did not undergo surgery for correction. And that is what my sister was telling me by phone—that Mom was going into surgery to treat the aortic dissection.

Hearing the news, I was in shock. It was very difficult to compartmentalize and put my daughter role down and think like a physician. Usually, I am able to do so, but that felt immensely different, primarily because I was in Denver and not at the bedside, and it was "a big one," meaning a life-threatening injury. Mom always said she wanted to go out with "the big one," and this certainly met the definition. Instead, she was going to have surgery.

In the preceding years, Mom underwent a few orthopedic surgeries, for which I was always there and even accompanied her into the operating room until she was properly sedated and the surgery began. Mom was sometimes nervous, so being a physician-daughter had its privileges. But this was different. Hearing about the extent of the injury and knowing that unless Mom had surgery she would die was difficult to comprehend. Mom had had angina before, perhaps even a mild heart attack, and she had a stent in one of her arteries. I had not been there for that cardiac event, and she did fine. I'd felt fine hearing about all of the earlier events, but the aortic aneurysm felt immensely different.

My siblings assured me that Mom had made the decision to undergo the surgery. Yet the three of us all felt bewildered by that, as the injury was technically "the big one" that Mom had always talked about. The one she was going to make her grand exit from this earth with. Well, not specifically that type of trauma—believe me, nobody wishes that type of vascular injury on *anybody*, because it is one of the most painful traumas to endure—but categorically an aortic aneurysm was the big one that would usher Mom to the other world for her to "be with Jesus," as she always said.

We three siblings discussed on the phone that Mom must have changed her mind, so we chose to not intervene on her decision. We would honor her wishes and support her in her choice of having surgery. To not have surgery was 100% fatal, in a matter of hours or perhaps a day or so. She could have comfort measures, we would be at her bedside, and she would peacefully pass. But that was not what was happening.

The surgery would be hours long. They would repair the aorta and, in the process, Mom would be placed into a deep, hypothermic state. Her heart would be stopped completely. That is beyond the bypass machine used to repair coronary arteries (arteries of the heart). In the deep hypothermic state, blood would be flowing, her body would be cooled, and, essentially, she would be in a suspended state, alive/ not alive. Technically, dead, and yet alive.

Her surgery was over ten hours long. Twenty-three minutes of those ten hours were spent in suspended animation, in deep hypothermia. She survived and was on a ventilator and sedated for thirty-six hours. During the thirty-six hours, she remained in the PACU, which is the super intensive care unit just outside the operating room.

People were notified, and everybody showed up to hold vigil at Mom's bedside. It was touch and go for thirty-six hours. No one knew what was going to happen. Vitals and labs and vigil, vitals and labs and vigil, that was the routine.

What happened next and for the next seven days outlines singularly the most difficult days and decisions in my life. Ever. It is very difficult to write about and yet is a necessary part of my story. It nearly killed me in the process—living it and then grieving, not the writing about it.

In Mom's case, a series of decisions were being made on parallel tracks. One track was we three siblings. The other track was the surgical team. As we three siblings discussed outcomes, next steps, short- and long-term decisions, we maintained Mom's perspectives and ideals and, moreover, her wishes as we knew them and as they were recorded in her appropriately filled-out end-of-life documents. They were all taken into consideration by us. What we kept passing around like an unknown object was the notion that Mom consented to this type of surgery. Instead, Mom could have been served with end-of-life measures, pain control, and then had a peaceful passing. As each of us examined the situation and decisions made, it just did not line up with what we knew about Mom. It did not seem to match Mom's convictions. We three, however, were on the same page: We agreed about Mom's next steps and care options. We were a team.

As the hours went by post-surgically, it was decided to wean Mom off the ventilator to see if she would breathe on her own. That was done, and she did not require breathing assistance, so she was extubated (breathing tube removed). Then she only needed oxygen by a mask. They lifted the sedation to see if she would come back into consciousness and she woke up. The doctors had feared that she would never regain consciousness and would "be a vegetable." That was distinctly not the case, but that was what I overheard as I stood behind the doctors when they were in conversation with one another in the hallway outside her room. They didn't think Mom had much of a chance. What they probably should have been fearing was that she would wake up. Mostly, however, I wanted her to wake up, so I could begin the process of saying goodbye.

Within a few minutes of Mom being conscious, she was alert, and speaking in a very weakened voice. She was asking what happened and attempting to wrap her mind around all that had occurred. She was both lucid and awake and that was totally surprising to both the surgeons and us as family. I am convinced the physicians thought she would never pull through the surgery, let alone come back into her right mind and be fully present.

Mom asked me if I knew what had happened to her. I replied by asking her what she thought had happened. (I was fully in physician mode by that time). Mom thought she had had a heart attack, and the surgery was to make the pain go away. I told her that was not true, that she did not have a heart attack. She was still in pain postoperatively, and it was the same type of pain she had experienced while in the ER but she also had pain all over her body as well. That was when I had an inkling that something did not seem as it was. Especially when I shared with her the diagnosis of the dissected aorta that extended down into both of her legs. When I explained that to Mom, she felt around and made the connection with the four chest tubes extruding from her body.

She said, "Wow. I never would have signed up for that surgery."

BOOM... mic drop.

But what actually dropped and went BOOM, was my heart, which fell out of my chest after it went up to my throat and then down again and I felt the wind leave me. I almost vomited.

Within ten minutes of being extubated and awake, Mom declared that she did not want to have had the surgery, and it was all too much and she could not recover and she wanted to go be with Jesus. She wanted to die. She no longer wanted to live. It was too much to overcome.

My Dilemma

What do you do when you hear those words, especially after that type of vascular injury and surgery? I'll tell you what you do. You listen to the patient, who will tell you their desired outcome in a situation. To be sure, I did press back a bit and ask Mom if she were to be able to recover would she want to live. She was firm. She did not think the injury was something she could overcome, nor did she want to overcome it. She just did not want to. She clearly felt that she could not. It was too much. She kept saying that she just wanted "to go to Jesus."

For the next six days, we sat vigil, talked with the surgical team, the ethics department, and close family. We were a tight circle as siblings and listened deeply to one another and honored one another throughout the entire time. And we honored our mom's wishes to "go home and be with Jesus." It was the hardest thing that I have ever negotiated, getting my mother off this planet.

The Process of Departure

The convictions and inklings that ensued over the six days post-injury and post-surgery included crucial conversations with surgeons, and confronting a medical system and decision process that never expected Mom to survive the surgery. In fact, they had never told her exactly what surgery she was going to have, nor did they obtain the proper informed consent. They did not set her up to survive the injury, as they did not perform the correct surgery. In addition to the aortic arch being repaired/replaced, they needed to repair the distal aortic injury by using a vascular surgical team. That team was never consulted. We were told there would be complications down the road post surgically and they would be dealt with *then*. That was not true. There was no intention to do so, no inclination to do so. The lead surgeon totally misunderstood my mom's convictions, requests, rights, and determination. He did not expect her to ever wake up.

We shielded Mom from all of that during those six days.

However, I think she had an inkling something was up, but she was in the active dying stage, so she was sorting through a lot. We never spoke to her of the difficulty we faced in getting her wishes accomplished, of the meetings we had, the stand-offs and the negotiating in defense of her wishes and decisions. Throughout the six days, we were isolated, triangulated, and manipulated by the physicians, the hospital, and the system, but we stood upon our convictions, as they were also Mom's convictions.

She had visitors who came to say goodbye and those who came to sit vigil. She even refused some visitors who came by. She wished my cousin a happy birthday, yes, on her actual birthday. And she gave a blessing to each of her children. She thanked each of us individually and spoke words of a lifetime in only a few phrases.

She was bringing closure to her eighty-three years. She was making her way. Each night I stayed with her, sleeping by her bed. When she needed something, I was there for her. Mainly, she wanted raspberry sherbet and ginger ale.

She was dying. Her labs showed it, her body began to show it, and the message of her soul and spirit were crystal clear. She let me know that she had seen Jesus and was ready to go. In the meantime, she needed more ice for her ginger ale and raspberry sherbet. So I raided all the ice machines and freezers I could get to in the middle of the night. Even now, when I drink anything cold, I simply ask quietly for more ice, more ice.

One of Mom's dying wishes was to get to a certain nursing home for her final days, which were actually her final hours. We moved heaven and earth to accomplish that for her. In the end, all that was available was what was considered a "male bed," meaning that, by census, a man was to take that nursing home bed, since they designated a certain number of beds available in a nursing home for males and females. So we used Mom's nickname of Hank, for Henrietta. We figured, why not?

Ultimately, Mom got a pass from the nursing home staff, because a particular nun had a soft spot for Mom and pulled some strings to accomplish Mom's wishes. Also, Mom had a handwritten note from the same nun, just in case Mom outlived the nun. The note stated that Mom could go to that particular nursing home. The note was her hall pass, as it were. A permission slip with divine endorsement.

Within one day of admittance to hospice and the desired nursing home, Mom's pain from the original aortic trauma was finally controlled and she passed peacefully from this earth. She was no longer suffering.

That was not true for me, however. Just under four months prior to Mom's passing, my father passed away. While I was not close to my father at the end of his life, I had, nonetheless, made the trek to his bedside and sat vigil with him as he prepared to depart this world, and it was impactful. But to lose Mom in such an unexpected way and with so much that we had to sort through while she was a patient took a right toll on me.

My Ongoing Dilemma

As a physician, I was faced with what I knew to be true about my mom's convictions and end-of-life choices. I had an inkling, which became more of a conviction, that the surgeons and the hospital really screwed up. I was convinced that Mom would have had a chance to live, and live relatively well, had they done the correct surgery. The recovery would have been long, arduous, and perhaps fraught with complications, but the way that Mom came out of the sedation was telling. It would take time—weeks, months, years—before I more fully understood what Mom was telling us in those moments and days between the surgery and her passing. Grief has a lot to say. It is a thing. It is a person. It is a place. Properly, it is a noun, and it is a proper Thing.

What nearly killed me was my inability to reconcile my inklings of Mom's convictions with my convictions. Mom's convictions were clear: She wanted her end of life to look a certain way, and that had been tampered with. It was my convictions that identified the various medical errors, exposing the physicians who had the lapses in judgment relative to a patient's decision-making and accuracy in the treatment/surgical plan—ultimately, what I saw as a betrayal of Mom's sovereignty as a patient. As a result, it was difficult to not want a different outcome than what had happened.

The "if only I had..." flag was flying full mast and with a strong headwind. I was convinced of my inklings all along of Mom's wishes being ignored and manipulated for what the surgeon wanted. Those inklings concretized into convictions and then became recalcitrant in my physical body and in my soul.

For the first year after Mom's passing, I could barely function. I went through the motions most days, then went home to hide out under the down feather comforter. I was grieving deeply, and I was suffering because I could not let the betrayal go. That impacted my mental, physical, and spiritual health. I dug deep into the hospital records to figure out the reason. The missteps were visible, and not within reason. They all seemed to bypass my mom's wishes, especially if one actually understood my mom's wishes. A partial surgery, and no ICU. The surgical plan and post operative plan did not match all of the life-saving measures that were needed—only about half of them. Recovery, in any way shape or form, requires all of those pieces to have been in place and completed. They simply were not. They were skipped over or not included at all.

My conclusion regarding Mom's treatment plan landed on the conclusion that it was what it was just because the surgeon chose so. He chose the surgery and omitted other parts, did not obtain additional consultants to participate, and did not choose to have Mom in intensive care post operatively. It would be against more odds than what should be been for Mom to even have a chance to recover. And with Mom waking up and being of sound mind post operatively, he for sure underestimated Mom, her children, and her decisions. He did not regard her sovereignty.

The completion of the first year without Mom segued into Covid and the lockdown. It was almost a year to the day that I contracted Covid and was ill enough to require hospitalization. The irony was that I was facing a big diagnosis on the anniversary of Mom's aneurysm. That was very telling. Grief had impacted my life, and my health and immune system took a major hit. I had a patient who had recently returned from Italy with "the weirdest bronchitis" I had ever seen. It was Covid and pneumonia. Who knew?! I was seemingly ground zero in Colorado with my diagnosis, as I was ill well before the lockdown occurred.

My Soul's Lessons

What I have come to understand by now, five years later, nearly to the day, is that Mom most likely had a great experience when she was in deep hypothermia, which cemented her conviction on where she wanted to go. Yes, from her perspective it would look daunting to her when faced with such a huge recovery challenge. She didn't cop out, give up, or quit.

She actively chose to move on to the next phase of her life, on the other side of the veil.

She shared with me at the end that she saw me and understood who I was. That had been a lifelong challenge in our relationship. She told me to "Go get 'em," meaning to live my life fully, as I am and as she saw and understood who I am. I can only gather that her insight about me came from the other side, as she did not possess or hold that perspective in our relationship until then.

I struggled with the what-ifs, especially as a physician. What if I had been in the ER? Would I have had different questions for the surgeon than my siblings? The answer was a clear hell, yes. But I don't second-guess either of my siblings. They did the very best they could and were just as bewildered about Mom's apparent decision as I was—we were, and remain, in one accord. They were unaware of what the surgeon was thinking or planning, but they were aware of Mom's wishes and felt the conflict therein.

What if I had spoken up when I overheard the surgeons talking and saying that they doubted Mom would ever would wake up? What if I created a lot more holy hell because Mom did not go to ICU after the PACU? Mostly, I did all those things. We, as Mom's children and advocates did all those things as we navigated her wishes and worked to honor her end-of-life choices. It was the hardest and most crucial week of my life, and it was very difficult to fight for her to be released, ultimately. In some ways you could say it was hell to get her to heaven.

Allowing for Grief

The conclusions I came to know some five years later were based upon more reflection and self-compassion. I know that I too did my very best for Mom, and while I do wish at times that things would have been different, that Mom would have had the correct surgery and recovery and that she would have lived more years, that was not for me to determine. She always wanted to outlive my father, and she did, by a smidgen. She faced many of her fears too. She had fears all along in her marriage, like what if she had to start over in life? She did have to do that, at age 55, and she built a beautiful life, established retirement and savings and investments. Things that she feared greatly, she overcame. Many fears she overcame. And she lived a full and fun life. Until the big one.

During Mom's visitation and funeral, my cousin's three-year-old daughter gave me a picture she had painted. She had been painting a lot with her grandma, my aunt. Lots of projects. Lots of pictures. All along, I inquired when I saw the various art projects if she had named them and what specifically the art pieces meant to her.

She always shared some of the names with me, and what meaning she saw in her artwork. So at Mom's visitation, when she gave me a picture she had painted for me, I asked her what the name of the painting was. She replied, *Swimming in Heaven.* I lost it, bawling my eyes out. You see, my mom had always been afraid of the water. That stemmed from an early childhood trauma where she nearly drowned. Throughout her life, she took swimming lessons, a lot of swimming lessons, at the local YWCA. The course was called Coward's Class, and Mom took it three times. While she passed each time, she never felt that comfortable in the water. Her whole life she wanted to conquer that fear and thus she made all of us kids take swimming lessons. We became prolific swimmers who love the water. Even just days before she had her aortic dissection, she was participating in water aerobics at the local workout facility. She and several other seniors were regulars. She was diligent to conquer her fears.

To receive that painting from a three-year-old who did not know the backstory about Mom and swimming was simply divine inspiration. A holy moment that we shared, knowing Mom was truly swimming in heaven.

Chapter 10
Epilogue to Trauma—My Soul's Journey

"You can never love another person unless you are equally involved in the beautiful but difficult spiritual work of learning to love yourself. There is within each of us, at the soul level, an enriching fountain of love. In other words, you do not have to go outside yourself to know what love is."
—John O'Donohue, *Anam Cara*

Going Deep into Presence and Anam Cara

Five years to the day after Mom's vascular trauma have now passed as I write this. It seems like only yesterday and a lifetime ago at the same time. As the days have marched by, I've thought to myself, *This is the longest time that I haven't seen my mom since I have been alive.* Most days are good, but grief can be a funny bugger; it catches you off guard, by a scent, a memory, a bluebird in the garden, a song, or a nudge. I believe all of the encounters that elicit a grief response are nudges from our loved ones. The veil is thin, very thin sometimes, and I can frequently sense my mom's presence and love.

She is well, and she has done more healing, not only in the physical world, but also in her soul and spirit. I get a sense of a reunion that she has had with loved ones, with my father, with her mom (my grandma) in particular. There is a peacefulness to her presence and a watchful eye and a push encouraging me on my journey as well.

A full circle has occurred in that she bore witness to my birth and I to her death. In the end, she gave a blessing to me by saying that she sees who I am, and to "go get 'em." It has taken time for me to see who I am after her passing. Part of the grief is finding who you are when both of your parents die. It feels as if you are an orphan, all grown up and little on the inside all at the same time.

I entered deep therapy just after the fourth-year anniversary of her passing. That season has born much fruit. I have been able to honor my grief, my life, and my strengths and weaknesses. I have reconnected with parts of my emotions and of my soul that were dissociated and fragmented. I have found a new way, which actually was the old way and the original way that I am able to relate to spirit, source, love, the divine. This connection to self is healing.

What seemed dormant for almost twenty-two years, which is technically an eleven-year cycle times two, has come alive in a new way in my life. By coming through a long season of grief, I too have entered a new way of living, on this side of the veil. I am coming home to who I actually have been my whole life. And I now understand that it was there all along. I was there all along. My beliefs were there all along. I too was on my soul's journey as well.

Seasons, Cycles, and Meaning

Cycles in our lifetime can be meaningful, if we reflect upon them and allow ourselves to be present with our feelings, thoughts, emotions, and processes. Eleven-year cycles, for me, represent a divine connection to the energy of creation, making eleven the most spiritually sensitive and intuitive of all numbers. The number twenty-two signifies that you have the strength to not only withstand life's adversities but also to transform them into opportunities for personal growth and spiritual development.

As I wrote earlier in the ceremony chapter, I have had two twenty-two-year cycles that were very meaningful. Within those cycles, there were mini-cycles, all bringing greater understanding, meaning, and connection in my life. Some parts of the cycles were just fucking hard; and I made it (you should see the other guy—ha).

The mystical has filled in my life (again), which I no longer resist. There is meaning in everything that has happened in my life. Many events, items, and occurrences turn out to be signs of divine guidance, encouragement, and awareness, but mostly Love. This is something that I have come to embrace.

Grief occupies a great space, properly so. I honor grief and all it has brought me and allowed me to experience. They say grief is the price of love. Okay, sounds good, and that is nice for a greeting card, maybe, but I see grief as the experience of change that then forever changes an individual, if we allow grief to have its way. If we resist grief, it is like trying to resist the rising tide or the wash of the flood. Water (grief) always has its way; it always wins.

Culturally, we don't grieve well, either as individuals or

collectively as a group. Platitudes are useless, avoidance is a disaster, and resistance is futile. But leaning into grief as in leaning into the wind can lift us and bring us higher into our sense of self, purpose, and life. But that is in its time, as you cannot hurry grief. You can't hurry the receding of the floodwaters. It just takes time.

For me, that time has been five years. I witness the space that grief has occupied in my life, I honor its presence, and I am ready to allow the ebbing of its tide so that I may continue my journey. Clinically, my experience would qualify as PTSD with a side dish of complex grief and condiments of anxiety traits with depressive features. Should you wonder, yes, I do know all the billing codes for those diagnoses. Happily, I will not submit them for reimbursement. Even more happily, I will allow them to begin to be part of my backstory versus my story. As my soul heals and the fragments meld, grief is not front and center. It is now softer and gentler and has faded more to the back of my being. It is there, I am aware, and I am at peace.

Grief's Complexity in My Journey

Since there was a significant amount of trauma regarding my mom's vascular injury, hospitalization, and death, it became difficult to work my way through the emotions, because they were entangled with so much complexity. Obviously, the trauma and the amount of pain my mom endured, the missteps of the surgical team, the betrayal of the hospital and medical system, and the gargantuan task of honoring my mom's legal and morally designed end-of-life choices should not have happened. That the dissection occurred, I grieve also, and I wished it never happened, but it did. But the other stuff was a right shit show. It would make sense that, rightfully so, some people would choose not to even look at the complexity, let alone work to understand and to unfold the emotions, the soul wounds, and the physical signs and symptoms of grief. Perhaps for some, that amount and type of grief would be an end-game for them. At times, it felt that way for me. Yet I submit that grief is part of the human condition and that I am not alone in this process. But working with that grief was both complex and difficult—and did I mention complex?!

Understanding My Journey

Here's what was interesting during a therapy session… coming onto the five-year anniversary of Mom's death, it felt a bit more poignant, perhaps because I'd had a year of intensive therapy and was facing some emotions I had avoided because I thought that if I faced them, I might never come back.

My emotions centered around letting my mom go and releasing her from this planet. While I had done that five years ago, I still felt tethered. I wasn't sure how to let go at the soul level. Ultimately, I learned this was a complex step due to the above-mentioned issues surrounding her vascular trauma and the shit show in the hospital. As a physician, that was particularly difficult for me to process, as I have helped several patients at their end of life with their choices, their autonomy, and their journey. Those events unfolded differently, without the level of betrayal and denial of the patient's choices that my mom experienced. What really was at the heart of Mom's trauma was her journey and her sovereignty as a patient, as a person, as a soul. That was violated at the deepest soul level, and yet the sovereignty of her soul prevailed. Mom's wishes were upheld, and she was allowed to leave this plane of living and go to the next step.

Intuition, Something We All Have

As a medical intuitive, I can see things. I have known this gift in my life's work as a physician for quite some time, and come to accept it. This gift shows up as images, words, ideas, perceptions, and shapes that bring me insight into communication and connection with my patients. I use it daily. But, with Mom, I couldn't *see* that part of her medical journey because of the trauma I had experienced around it. The trauma clouded my ability to discern what I was feeling. That is both normal, and a direct result of trauma.

For us to better understand: Trauma is what happens inside us, in our body, in our spirit, in our soul. It is in response to experiencing a traumatic event. In turn, the traumatic event is what happened to Mom as her aorta ruptured and in the subsequent surgery and less-than-necessary medical care and support. That occurred to her and to me as a person who lost their mother. It was the trauma, however, that had me in its clutches. My soul was held captive by the traumatic events that caused a trauma response inside of me. Many parts of me were in shutdown, survival mode. Disconnected on the inside, and fragmented within my very being.

That was my exact point of suffering. I couldn't *see* how or why Mom's will had been so strongly disregarded and why we had to fight so hard to reinstate her end-of-life wishes. I believed that if I could see and understand, I could then be free and heal. Truthfully, at some level, I wished she had received the correct surgery so perhaps she would still be alive. I missed my mom. I wanted her to live longer than she did.

While all of that seemed reasonable, without therapy I couldn't reconcile it at all. The trauma effect in my body, soul, and spirit was present, and I was suffering as a result.

Healing Souls by Connecting with My Intuition

As previously mentioned, my therapist does not leave a stone unturned. In fact, those were her words as we entered the hallowed space of held emotions, with its somatic features, during a particular therapy session.

As I opened to the event of Mom being in the hospital, it occurred to me to view those events from Mom's perspective. As I did that, a transcendence occurred. I was on another plane. I was observing the traumatic events from a deep listening perspective and, in doing so, I believe the realm of the soul and spirit opened. There were both souls, my mom's and mine. I felt as if a veil was lifted and I could see the medical team surrounding Mom. She was not only fully sedated but also in a deep hypothermic state. That is the state of suspended animation—death, not death, death. That was where Mom most likely got her view of the other side. Truth be told, she *was* on the other side, and she had to come back after those twenty-three measured minutes, back from timelessness to time. That is most likely the reason why she awoke with such conviction about wanting to go be with Jesus and not be on the earth anymore.

Okay, that made sense to me. As I saw that from my transcendent state during the therapy session, my body connected with the experience and I could feel the trauma releasing from my fascia, tissues, heart, and soul. My questions were being so sublimely answered a peaceful rest that began to fill my being. I was connecting at the soul level and time felt suspended during that process of deep observation. I was fully present, yet on a different plane.

What happened next was surprising. I could *see* my mom's soul and its sovereignty. It was like a force—waves of love, strength, and power. It wasn't scary at all. In fact, it was peaceful, steady, and assured. It had chambers and restful spots, and it was quiet and strong. There were shadow areas and areas with soft lighting and a glow. Then I could see that there possibly was a discussion, a decision, or some type of pause that occurred when Mom was in deep hypothermia. The surgeons paused to check their work, and I have an inkling that they wondered about doing more, or perhaps were rethinking their decisions. But what came to be so very clear was that the sovereignty of Mom's soul said, *This is enough. No matter what, I am not coming back. No matter what, I am ready to go, to leave this earth and not return.* It did not seem that the surgeon was aware of that soul's presence and determination other than he made the decision to not change the direction of the surgical process, thus establishing the trajectory of Mom's inability to recover. On some level, he appeared beset or perhaps bewildered with his decisions, given the appearance of the surgical field he was in while performing the operation.

I recalled my thinking in real time from five years ago. I remembered knowing that Mom was in surgery, marking the hours of her surgery, imagining what was transpiring while I was still in Colorado awaiting my flight to Michigan. I remember saying over and over, "It's okay if you go, Mom. I understand. We all understand." It was not clear that she would survive the surgery, that uncertainty was very strong. Her prognosis was grave and, in those moments, and at that time, I did release her. What choice did I have? She was hanging by a thread and who knew the outcome?

Five years later, still in my grief, it was my trauma connecting with her trauma, and it was the holding of that joint trauma and joint suffering that allowed for the clarity of vision, of understanding, as to where Mom's decisions came from when she awoke post-surgically. Then, as her children, we had to face all the challenges that followed, in light of her wishes, and it was just so very hard to get her dying wishes upheld.

It felt like a spiritual and soul-driven whiplash I experienced while she was unconscious. I was doing everything I could to hold her on the planet and then, with her waking up from the surgery and being so sure about departing the earth, I had to pivot 180 degrees to begin to hold her in such a way as to release her off the planet. That process was what created a lot of traumas in my body, especially through the nervous system, fascia, and musculoskeletal system. I hurt all over. Trauma was racking up points and my body was keeping the score. I experienced physical changes in my root chakra, where survival is held, in the lower back, pelvis, hips. All of that was obvious when looked at retrospectively. At the time, though, and for subsequent years, I was miserable, with variations on the theme.

What became clear in that particular therapy session, however, five years later, was how very clearly Mom's sovereignty came through in her choices during her surgery. Her outcome was driven by her soul, and the physicians went along with her sovereignty, most likely at a subconscious level. That is a bit mysterious and mystical. Yet her soul's sovereignty was leading the way, even if we all were too traumatized, too conditioned, or too unconscious to understand it at the time.

Healing of Body and Soul

What was witnessed some five years later by deep observation and intuition was both mystical and mysterious, and it was beyond beautiful. The experience provided understanding, context, and, therefore, meaning around the traumatic event. You see, Mom never liked the medical system and always wanted to beat the doctors at their game. She wanted her care on her terms. Seeing her soul in the moment of reflection, of transcendence, in that therapy session, seeing the mystery of her soul fully at work, assured me that no matter what anyone did or would try to do, her soul's decision had taken the lead and determined her outcome.

On seeing that, my whole body went into a state of relaxation and release. There weren't tears, but rather a deep, abiding peace, release, and then more peace. It was beautiful, amazing, as my suffering was also released and I was healing too. My low back, hips, fascia, and nervous system all began what could be described as an unwinding. Stretching and moving became much less painful. The trauma was being released from my body, and my body was free to catch up with my soul's healing. Mom was healed and I was healing. That deep observational experience was what allowed me to fully let my mom go, after five years. I could clearly see it was her soul that had made the decisions, after all. No matter what.

What an amazingly beautiful experience and concept. The mystery of the soul is wondrous. I was in a state of both awe and wonder. The soul is an amazing concept. It is a thing.

Common Humanity in Our Experiences

As a physician and a person, I know that we all experience grief. Understanding that concept has allowed me to come into greater self-compassion and then connection back to myself, my higher Self, and my source of love, spirit, and the

Universe in a very special way. Grief and finding meaning has led me back home to myself. I embrace who I am and know that the path I am on is meant to be traveled, and perhaps even be a travelogue. Those five years were not wasted, nor was my life waylaid. I was simply healing and growing and transforming from what that massive change had brought to my life.

My Soul's Lessons

The Mystic and Wounded Healer experiences both trauma and healing in life, experiences that are meant to be shared. Traumatic events can often be seen as gifts. Healing from traumatic events and the traumas stored in the body is my work now. This is different from just being a physician (as if being a physician isn't enough already… *wink*). It is enough, I have done enough, I have been enough, I have healed enough, and I am enough. And now I move into a new phase of my life to bring healing to others from a deeper well, a different place, and with the support of the other world(s).

My spiritual journey is now opened into a more Celtic tradition of seeking, worshiping, and understanding a very old tradition that honors the spirit in everything. Everything has a spirit and is alive. Additionally, taking my healing journey further will include studying shamanic work within the Celtic traditions. This is where my intuition, my inklings, are taking me. This is where my soul feels the freest; not cultured, but free, wild, and open. This is where my life has always led me. I have not missed out. I have been on this path all along. Now I embrace it even more. And I am grateful.

The push from my mom, her end-of-life encouragement to me—I get it now. I know what she meant and what I am meant to do. It took a while, and that's okay. Nothing was wasted, ever. So now I choose to live my life in a way to honor her life and my own soul's sovereignty by fully embracing who I am meant to be, understanding all along that my soul knew that and fully intended it to be this way. And so it is.

Chapter 11
Ceremony Number Two

"Self-healing is easier said than done, and yet it is within each person's power. Sometimes, it is the very thing that wakes you up to yourself and your own powers."
—Colleen Deatsman, *The Hollow Bone*

Prologue to Ceremony Two (Circa 2024)

What I did not realize at the time took various twists and turns throughout the next twenty-two years to understand: I never left God, Spirit, Source, or Love. We can't, because they are everywhere and in everything. Spirit, source, and love essentially permeate everything. It is only our awareness of them that alters our perception, but they are always there.

What I was leaving when I left the church was a set of beliefs, a dogma, doctrine, teaching, and people who believed a certain way. And not the way I believed. But I never left God and God never left me... *ever*. Actually, I took God with me, as I continued to seek truth through a greater understanding of love and connection.

During the past twenty-two years, I have been a truth-seeker. Anywhere there was truth, love, and a life centered in that belief, I was all in. There were no dogma or diatribes, no attendance or demands on my beliefs, life, time, or commitments. I was free to believe how I wanted, and I wanted the root belief of Love as the center for all things; I wanted the belief that God/spirit/source is everywhere, in everything, and permeates all of life. Connecting to self and to source brings life and liberty in all areas. If that was blocked or impeded, then I worked to figure out why. Or just walked away. It was that simple.

I read books and attended seminars on contemplative prayer, Celtic teachings, Buddhist teachings, and the Church of Light in Boulder, Colorado, where I was trained as a psychic and provided with a minister's certificate. I was mentored by other physicians who were striking out on their own creative paths. Often, they had left medicine for a more personal calling and life's work. That felt true to me, but not the leaving medicine part. I continued to practice, as I loved being a physician, a healer, but I was frustrated with health-care in America. Being a physician was not the same as being a healer. More and more, I was being called into the intuitive work, into mental health and a mind/body/spirit approach to care. It permeated everything, just like Love did. Not a coincidence, I decided. It was my path. And I was on it.

I read anything and everything that supported my beliefs, and left everything else alone. I had read enough of the "only way to heaven" perspective. I wasn't interested in praise and worship, did not care who was lord, and did not have any remaining fucks to fly regarding any kind of kingdom established here on earth. Full stop. It was hard core. I felt it, I lived it. That affected my relationships, choices, and perspectives. I was boundaried up and it was a strong no man's land that no one could traverse. I was recalcitrant.

Here's the fly in the ointment... I had a bit of confusion regarding how it played out, which stemmed from my wounding and hurts that led to the subsequent disconnection from myself. A dissociation of my own mind, body, and spirit.

As a physician, my training in trauma-informed care has been deep and continuous, and a main portion of my ongoing learning as a physician. Gabor Maté is one of my mentors. His work is seminal regarding trauma, dissociation, and addictions. One thing he said changed my world, my approach to life, and my approach to treatment with patients. He stated that, "All trauma causes us to disconnect from ourselves. It is not perceived as safe to be connected. So we disconnect."

If we disconnect enough, we leave the planet—we make a choice to not continue to live here. If we remain on earth, yet disconnected, there is a tether between our higher self and our disconnected self. This is where addictions, dysfunctional behaviors, and other behaviors are used as tools to maintain as much connection as we can tolerate.

That idea profoundly changed my paradigm of care, and I saw bad habits, behaviors, and addictions as a way to remain attached to ourselves. Despite the often destructive outcomes, at least we were still connected, at some level. That rocked my worldview and spiritual view, and infused hope to so many patients I worked with. It changed their lives. It changed my life.

I believe this tether, this attachment, is mediated by our soul. Here is where our soul does its work. It is not only about mental health and therapy and behavior modification, but/and our soul works in this area to mediate between our spirit and body. We cannot heal our mental health without healing our soul and our body, as we are intricately intertwined.

There is an entire area of study and treatment regarding attachment disorders; or another way to look at it is disordered attachment. The goal in that therapy is to find safety through attachment, primarily by understanding the attachment to safe people, i.e., parents, family, etc. This allows us to safely navigate and neuroregulate through life each day.

What I learned and, moreover, what I experienced, was that in order to connect with others, I first needed to connect or reconnect with myself. From there, I could go anywhere, since I was connected to my higher self (spirit), soul, and body. I could navigate life because I was connected first to myself and then to others. *Myself* becomes the anchor. Home base.

Our soul is not in us, but surrounds us, envelops us. It is suffused with our body and spirit. It is eternal, and we have many iterations as the soul learns and grows and becomes. It is mysterious, secret, and sacred and includes shadow and light. It is altogether holy and hallowed ground. I learned that the prophetic is not about telling the future, but rather a call to return to the ancient roots of our far-back people, our ancestors. There are no dogma, doctrine, rules, or regulations to follow. Rather, we follow the echo of our soul. A response inside of us to the call from spirit inside and beyond us. Intimate and afar.

That was the pull I felt all my life. That was the tether that held me, in addition, to the tether of the dissociative behaviors as I fully had a human experience. I was experiencing the tether of the call, the pull between souls and between creator and souls, my soul.

My human behaviors on the tether were not always supportive of healthy living. I had given up on some lifestyle choices, did not exercise as much, did not eat wholesome foods (mostly). I opted for convenience. I opted for junk food, drank more alcohol, worked very hard, and felt stressed. Because, honestly, I was wounded. I was still hurting. In the twenty-two years since the first ceremony, and despite seeking and living my truth, a lot of life happened. I was disconnected, dissociated, and—in some parts of myself—at war with myself. I had been diagnosed with autoimmunity and chronic fatigue, with recalcitrant inflammation. My body was suffering. Parts of my soul needed healing. My body was aching for healing. I was a physician, and I couldn't figure out how to heal, despite my best efforts. Shame, shame.... Then there's that too! (Eye-roll.) I needed help.

I had experienced business successes and failures, financial ruin, deaths of friends and family—some sudden, some expected. Ups and down of the economy. Changes in healthcare and jobs. Pandemics, illness, and a near-death experience for myself.

It. All. Took. A. Toll.
And I needed... help.

Bardos

In the year after my mom died suddenly, unexpectedly, at the hands of a highly dysfunctional medical system, I was barely hanging on. The tether was long and did not feel very strong. While I did not have any suicidal ideation, I did not have a strong determination either.

Bardos, I was in the bardos.

Pause for a definition:

- Bardos: "In Tibetan Buddhism, the bardos are the intermediate states of existence between death and rebirth. The word 'bardo' is a Tibetan word that translates to 'gap, interval, intermediate state, transitional process, or in between.'" —Andrew Holecek

- Bardos: "The concept of the bardos can also be applied to other periods in life when the normal way of life is suspended, such as during an illness or meditation retreat. These periods can be beneficial for spiritual progress, but they can also present challenges." —Wikipedia
- Bardos: "The state of the soul between death and rebirth." —Dictionary.com

All of Those Were True

As I paddled around in the bardos, as I walked, sat, prostrated, and often felt bewildered, I also sought truth. I sought healing and studied trauma and its effect on the body, soul, and spirit.

Grief had its way with me and, over time, I came through.

Four years after Mom passed, I chose to go into deep therapy. Two types: grief therapy and gestalt somatic therapy. The grief therapy helped me understand that it would still take time and to allow grief in its many faces to have its space and place in my life after the loss of my mother changed me in a fundamental way. I simply wasn't the same afterward. The gestalt therapy was new, but made sense. It was a holistic view of therapy. The somatic-based therapy would address the trauma that was recalcitrant in my body and soul.

Psychotherapy is taught, learned, and researched. Therapists are good and not so good. Medicine is taught, learned, and researched. Physicians are good and not so good. My goal was to find both a good therapist and a good team of physicians to help me heal.

It was the gestalt somatic emotional therapy that had some of the biggest impacts upon my life. My holistic cardiologist and integrative osteopathic family physician help me with my physical health. My heart was wounded, literally. I had palpitations, paroxysms of atrial fibrillations, and some mild to almost moderate coronary artery disease. My weight was out of control and metabolically I was imbalanced. I required supplementation, medication, and testing. Fortunately, my physical health has been responding and recovering. I am grateful for my medical team. They see me and hear me and stand with me for healing. They are amazing. I am recovered.

As for my mental health, the grief and dissociation and wounding of my soul is healing. This work has been a big lift and requires focused effort by both me and my therapist. Hours of sessions, plus the self-imposed homework of writing, contemplation, and Self Compassion & Connection™ protocol and reading. I really felt that my wounding and healing were not a random life path. Rather, by identifying with the Wounded Healer archetype, my life, story, and experience would help me and many others heal. I was understanding that through arriving at the definition of a Wounded Healer, through describing my journey and healing, and not by trying to identify with an outward idea or set of beliefs. Also, I did not bypass anything to get here. My therapist made sure of that. Ahem... thanks! I faced it all.

In this process, I arrived at lap nine of ten of my therapy and I wanted out. I felt done. Therapy was over, and I was cured. My therapist said, "Okay. Well, with where you are, you can live an amazingly full and complete life with the work you've done. But if you want, you can go a bit more and see if there are any more gems that await you." Ah, the teaser.

Without hesitation, I was in. I want all the gems. Take no prisoners, leave no bounty.

I realized that, at the time, I was experiencing the collective fatigue I had been carrying since the baby-and-bathwater ceremony and way before then. The wounding was deep and pervasive. The upside was that the healing could be deep and pervasive as well. I wanted to be done with the struggle to regain my physical health, and I wanted healing. I wanted all of it. After all, I believed that I should not be exempt from receiving the same benefit of my body's inherent capacity to heal and the results of the Self Compassion and Connection™ I had developed. Healing and truth were what I was seeking.

So I looked back at the first ceremony and saw the truth and the shadow. I saw that when I threw out the religion and kept my faith and truth, I looked to settle scores but aimed at the wrong enemy. I fought my body. I fought parts of my soul and spirit. In making strong boundaries, some parts of me were left on the other side, pretty much in no man's land. They were there, but detached—kinda like a closet or room full of things both precious and not so precious, but where I did not have the ability to open the door to access the room. That pulled on me and weighed on my life, physically, and I fought it. I fought myself and, in doing so, my body responded with inflammation and autoimmunity from the disconnection. To be sure, I am not laying blame on myself for all my ailments and illnesses. There were a lot of infections and traumatic events that I had experienced. However, can there be lessons from them? Yes, I believe so. If we choose to want to know. And I did.

As a physician, I see how this feels a bit in the mystery part of being human. There are certain things in medicine that appear linear: a person inverts their ankle coming down from a basketball rebound and sustains a sprain or fracture to their ankle. But it is in the area of autoimmunity, chronic illness, and multiple illnesses combined where the central dysfunction seems to be in the psycho-neuro-endo-immune system. That system runs through our fascia, which literally encompasses and envelops every part of our being. Sounds kinda soulish to me. Just sayin', it all resonated very strongly for my healing and restoration of my soul and for my life's work.

For that reason, I arose early on the morning of the Snow Moon and began my Celtic shamanic drumming and burning bowl ceremony two. I wanted change. I wanted the fight with myself to be done. I understood cognitively, collectively, wholly, and I wanted to be on the other side of it.

I wrote down on packaging paper all that I wanted to see burn, then I mixed it with other packaging paper and kindling wood. I had already established my altar outside in my backyard the day before. I felt led to have rose quartz, a Madonna, our first labradoodle's paw print, red pine branches, pinecones, and maple tree sticks. I used a buffalo hide drum (recorded music) and wooden matches.

I faced east to the pre-dawn sky with gratitude and anticipation. Thanking my ancestors, guides, mentors, spirits, and all who would choose to witness the ceremony, I called them in. The match was struck and held to the paper. *Woosh.* The flames took off and within a few short minutes, the pile of paper, kindling, pine needles, and oak leaf was reduced to ash. I then gave thanks and spread the ashes on the altar that would remain in place until the full moon passed.

My Soul's Lessons

The ceremony was complete. The fight was over. I would begin anew, rising from the ashes to live again, in a new way. I was at peace. The clarity that ceremony provided allowed me to see how I had always deferred to others and often felt envious of other people's success, regretful of my failures and tribulations. Not ever finding the "there" I was aiming for, I realized the "there" is "here." Home is within me, true north, and the way inward was the way forward. The powers that others saw in me were there. I needed to believe it myself. I needed to accept that truth and allow all of those skills, gifts, and talents—essentially, my power—to come through my life. No more shutdown survival mode. Rather, being open and going forward and trusting that I knew the way because I had done the inward work.

I was at home in the trees, the old bed of Lake Michigan, and within my own body and soul. At last, I had arrived. And. It. Felt. Good.

The End

But not really. Stay tuned for my next book...

Appendix

There is no appendix.*

*It is missing because I had the remnants of my appendix removed after it ruptured. The physician surgeon who saved my life in October 1973 at Butterworth Hospital, Grand Rapids, Michigan, was Peter Hayes, MD. He was a kind soul and a true healer. Thank you.

Resources

Medical care, health coaching, true self-directed healing, and curated health and wellness education can be gathered at drmarylouder.com.

Dr. Mary Louder Courses

- **My Anxiety Code**™—Anxiety as a messenger, not a diagnosis. Find your Unique Code. A masterclass to learn from.
- **The Hero's Genome**™—A curated course on genomics. Become the hero of your own health journey.
- **HEAL™**—A program for those who desire a journey of hope, healing and wholeness.
- **The Neural Resilience Method™**—A method of recovering from trauma and gaining resilience for your next steps of healing. A neural transformative process.

Recommended Books

- *Atlas of the Heart*, by Brené Brown.
- *The Hollow Bone*, by Colleen Deatsman.

Acknowledgments

This work would not be complete without the love, support, feedback, input, and shared work and lives of many people. *My tribe*, as I affectionately call them. Here they are, in no specific order, but not really random, either...

Andy Louder—My true love, sounding board, and partner in this life.

Sophie Louder—Our first labradoodle, who taught me so much. I love you! Namaste.

Lucy Louise Linder-Louder—Eye-roll on the name (her idea to include her whole name). Our present and accounted for labradoodle, an extraordinary critter, embodied and full of life!

Grace Kerina—My editor and a true book whisper. Thank you.

Henrietta Zoe Fegel-Mark—My mother. Thank you. I live your legacy.

Joe Mark, Sr.—My father. I wish peace for your soul.

Grandma Louise Schurk-Fegel—My namesake, and a true first love of mine. You saw me and knew me from day one. Even before that.

The Sister Marie Goretti Prayer Group—My mom's tribe (aka, The Clubski). They welcomed me on the day of my birth, in Butterworth hospital. Thank you for teaching me to party from day *one*! And for the back-scratcher for Mom's stitches too!

Joe Mark, Jr.—My big brother. I know you are watching out for me, as all big brothers do.

Karol Mark-Tiemersma—My sister. Our family was complete when you showed up. You have been worth the extra plate.

Leah Sheffield-Boden—The English girl who arrived in Michigan for a summer and left as a friend for life. Sharing cuppas, daily knock-ups, ba-A-con, Olgies, and Amy Grant.

Shyamaa Creaven PhD—Anam Cara. Gratitude, so much gratitude, to be together—again.

Jill Steinbrener-Olson—You are welcome, for all my help during college and, of course, the black walnut cookies! A friend for generations.

Mary Finch-Steele—My 23 and Me cousin, a true surprise gift. 23 and WTF?! xo from "Go to hell Mary."

Alecia Beth Moore-Hart (aka P!NK)—You. Helped. Me. Heal. Thank you!

Brené Brown, PhD—Your work has transformed my life and my work. You are a soul-sister from a different mister and mom!

UL and AMK—Thank you for your support, and I wish you both peace for the journey.

Cindy Morris—A teacher, mentor, and friend. Thank you for your support in my "young 'un" days.

Kristen Neff, PhD—Thank you for your work and the self-compassion that I have learned from you.

Gabor Maté, MD—Thank you for sharing your work and your wisdom. I use it in your honor.

May Erlewine—Michigan's treasured folk musician and my podcast music provider. Thank you!

The many other musicians to whom I listen—Thank you. You feed my soul, continually!

John O'Donohue—Your life and writings inspire my Soul. Thank you.

Sarah Bamford-Seidelmann, MD—A true healer and creative shaman. Thank you for your encouragement, writing class, editorial referral, and the healing work you bring to the world.

To Nature Itself, the Universe, and God with all Its wisdom and insight—Anam Cara.

About the Author

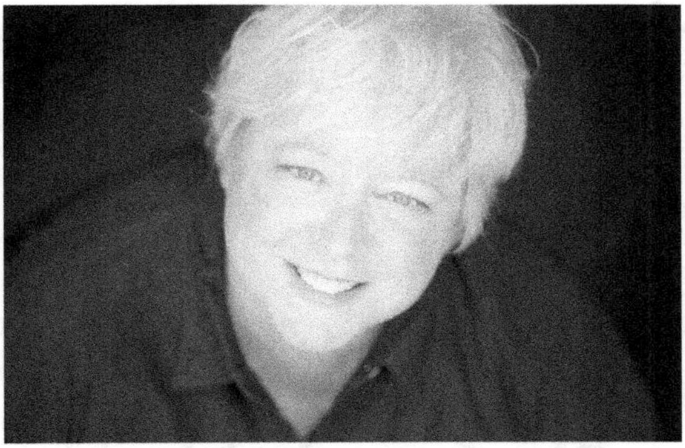

Mary Louder, DO, was born and raised in Grand Rapids, Michigan. She is a graduate of Northview High School, the University of Montana, and Michigan State University College of Osteopathic Medicine. She completed her internship and residency through Michigan State University at Lansing General Hospital (no longer there) and St. Mary's Hospital in Grand Rapids.

She has lived in three different states: Michigan, Montana, and Colorado. Now she and her family reside just east of the shore of Lake Michigan. She is an avid bike rider, swimmer, and walker in the woods (not a hiker; just an ambler). She loves to collect rocks, read, watch British crime shows, and listen to a variety of music. She is an avid cook and a pretty damn good baker.

Mary's clinic is in Holland, Michigan, and can be found

online at drmarylouder.com. Her work includes patient care, and mentorship to physicians and other health care providers. Currently, she is developing learning modules and retreats for people who wish to experience the HEAL program through The Self-Compassion and Connection™ pathway and The Neural Resilience Method™ with the felt sense of self-healing. You can find details on her website.

Mary's podcast is *Since You Put It That Way* and can be found on Apple, Spotify, YouTube, and Buzzsprout, or wherever you listen to your podcasts. You can also find, follow, and subscribe to her YouTube channel (@drmarylouder) and her LinkedIn (@drmarylouder).

Chapter 12
Here Comes Saturn, Again—Learning, Unlearning, Relearning

Full Circle, Again

P!nk, the musician, epic performer, and powerful badass was in town. The town was Missoula, Montana, a city and community paramount in my formation as a young adult. Hell, Missoula was formative for me as an older adult as well. From that adulting, I also had some undoing to do. My friend Jill (a fifth generation Missoulian and my favorite GRIZ person) says she saw a sign in Europe that said: "Learn, Un-learn, Re-learn." Seems about right. Ironically, she traveled to Europe for a sign, and I went back to Missoula for mine.

In the summer of 2024, I turned sixty-two years old. I was born in 1962, so that made 2024 a special birthday, which is given a few name variations: *platinum*, like my hair; and a Beddian birthday, which is when someone turns the same age as the year they're born. That once-in-a-lifetime occurrence is named for New York firefighter Bobby Beddia, who made the birthday observation and, according to a story in *The New Yorker*, was thrilled to reach the milestone himself at 53. He, unfortunately, was later killed in the line of duty as a first responder.

My birthday that year also coincided with the August super, blue, full moon. It was also on the tail of my *second* Saturn return. In Western astrology, a first Saturn return occurs around age 28-30 and has the following psychological characteristics: a time of reaching adulthood and facing adult responsibilities for the first time. It can be a time of confrontation, confusion, and fear, but it can also be an invitation to step into purpose, individuality, and authentic expression.

A second Saturn return is believed to occur between the ages of 58 and 60, and can extend two and a half years, plus or minus a year either side. It's a time when a person is said to cross over a major threshold and enter the next stage of life: maturity. This is when a person is planning their retirement, which is considered the second major transformative time of their life. It's also a time to move into more of a mentorship role, offering wisdom to those entering their first Saturn return.

Saturn is known as the teacher of the zodiac, and when it returns to the degree in its orbit occupied at the time of a person's birth, it's said to be schooling that person. The person is said to learn what behaviors and actions are no longer in line with their vision for the future, and to be shown the right path. This can lead to internal conflicts, among other things, as the universe is said to be urging the person to shed people, situations, and behaviors that are no longer working for them.

It would be like that phrase and picture that we commonly see as a meme: Me at age 30 (which is the first Saturn return). And now how is it was going? Me at age 61 (which is the second Saturn return). Rightfully so, I am thankful for an extra opportunity of the second Saturn return so that I may hit the mark of the many things that perhaps I was a bit slow on the uptake about prior to this time. And then to share my wisdom, knowledge, and experience. In turn, I am thankful for those who have shared their wisdom and experience with me.

Whew, that was a few paragraphs of saying it was an epic trip to Missoula, Montana, at an epic time in my life. As it went, I found that a lot of adjustments were needed that required extra planning. There were changes in the traveling and lodging plans, and then even for the dates and the period of time while traveling, everything that was planned had to be adjusted, planned, and planned again. It was a bunch of moving parts, all beyond one's control. A time to go with the flow and ride the wave. As a result, I had to work to stay connected to myself or "in my body." Typically, when I went on vacation, I would unwind and the travel plans worked, and that was that. Not this time, but that all played a part in the unfolding of my understanding and was a part of the journey.

Knowing that I was finishing this memoir, it felt right to head to the Mansfield Library on the University of Montana campus and tap into the quiet, studious atmosphere of creating. That writing day came after I attended the P!nk concert held at the Washington-Grizzly football stadium. A sold-out crowd, an epic venue, and full-circle moments were experienced on several issues.

Here is some insight on one of them... as a freshman at UM, I became religious in an attempt to belong. I did not trust myself to not be too wild; therefore, getting some religion might be a good thing. Perhaps a little bit of religion might have gone a long way, but instead, I jumped in with both feet and had a whole life conversion. My decades-long experiences in religion became a major Learning, Unlearning, and Relearning in my life.

What I learned while being a new convert was that music

was mostly of the devil, so I smashed my albums—all of them. I had some really classic ones too. It was a thing back in the eighties that if you played an album backward, you might hear a hidden satanic message. While that never happened in my experience, I nevertheless smashed my album collection. Then, some forty years later, there I was back on the same campus where I had ritualistically smashed my albums, going to a P!nk concert.

At the concert, I took a deep breath and went quiet on the inside to connect with the moment and event and venue. Then it struck me: I had never needed to smash my albums to belong. The smashing of my personal items became a metaphor. I never needed to destroy who I really was to fit in. Rather, I'd given myself away in order to belong. I was no longer up for negotiation. The many things I did to belong caused me to leave who I really was at my core—a wonderful, caring, generous, wise soul who often showed up and frequently had something to say from a unique perspective. Granted, the unique perspective was often provided with some cheekiness and salty humor, but nonetheless was genuine and authentic to who I was.

That was the very point about me that people seemed challenged by and that was, starting from when I was young, reinforced over time. It led to the maladaptive behavior, stemming from the backstory, biology, and biography that I adopted to fit in. All along, I wanted to belong, I wanted to figure out what I was meant to be and do, as I was sure it was something cool that I would be head over heels for.

At somewhere around 61-and-a-half years of age and attending the P!nk concert, I realized I was who I was always meant to be. Sitting in that stadium singing my heart out, jumping up and down declaring, "I AM HERE" with thirty-thousand-plus other individual souls, it solidified. I had turned the needed corners in my belonging and my sense of becoming. I had arrived. I was home.

The work I am doing as a physician includes mentorship, writing, educating, and influencing our next generation of physicians and patients. The way I perceive and see things is just fine, and it is different than most other physicians, and that is okay. I am grateful to know that, all along, I never needed to give up part of myself to be myself and to live out what may be considered my calling.

Thank you, P!nk (Alecia Beth Moore-Hart). Your music and your message have brought healing to my soul. And Missoula, the University of Montana, my family, and friends in and around Missoula. Thank you.

Along life's way, people, homes, addresses, jobs, and projects have come and gone. Sometimes things concluded organically, with grace, and sometimes things and circumstances were blown to smithereens. Either way, I was out, and it was over, but occasionally I had to mop and clean or do rescue and recovery. It all depended.

Over time, between my first and second Saturn returns, I learned that I had some early patterning of decision-making and some distressful events that led me to conclude relationships or circumstances in a not so good way, as I did not feel safe, seen, or understood. Now I understand that it is safe to be who I am, it is safe to be seen and to be exactly who I am.

People will do things differently than me and that is okay. Perhaps people even do things *to* us versus *with* us. Their behavior comes from their own early experiences, distressful or healthy, and typically people are unaware of their impact upon another in what may be considered a traumatic way. In turn, my response(s) now, after a significant amount of healing, therapy, and self-compassion, show that I've learned that I may live in and from a safe place, with boundaries and self-compassionately driven guidelines for my physical, mental, emotional, and spiritual health.

Today, sitting in the library on the University of Montana campus, I see all of the young students (they get younger each year) and I think of how they have their whole lives in front of them. So many things they don't even know yet will come their way. And I sit among them, understanding that life, with all its winding roads, leads us to exactly where we need to be.

I am grateful for my many experiences and my lessons. I am glad Saturn came 'round again, allowing me to have many full-circle moments. I look ahead to my third Saturn return at 88 years old. They have gotten better each time. Next time should be beyond *epic*! Full circle....

My Soul's Lessons

The Universe, Love, God, Source (you pick, please) is a friendly place. Signs, omens, and experiences can propel me forward in the way that I am meant to live. Returning to the UM campus where I had put so many stakes down in the ground was liberating. Getting to see P!nk in concert, was a sign, an omen. Participating in her concerts (which you can do by singing at the top of your lungs) was the icing on the cake of a second Saturn return.

My soul's loose ends were more connected, things made sense, and the clarity for the next steps in my journey solidified. Mostly, I was able to celebrate all that I had been through, and celebrate that I was able to return to a place I greatly loved, with my great love, and share all of it with him. It was very sweet indeed.

Chapter 13
The Way Inward Is the Way Forward

"The safest place to be is connected to yourself. From there, you can go anywhere."
—Mary Louder, DO

Self-Compassion and Connection™ and a Felt Sense

What I have learned, accepted, and begun practicing fully is an embodied approach to medical care. Am I a healer? Yes. Do I prescribe medications? Yes, when needed. Do my patients need surgery sometimes? Yes. Are there spontaneous remissions and rapid healings without relapses? Yes, any or all the above. Wait, do some of the patients die? Yes, because eventually we all die. Just like with bleeding—eventually all bleeding will stop. Can an ultimate healing be a release into the unseen realm of the next life? Yes, probably technically that happens all the time, yes. But first and typically foremost, people get their lives back, though it is not usually the same life they started with pre-illness, pre-diagnosis, and pre-treatment. It is, by and large, a life more in line with their true purpose and reason for being. It is their authentic life. That is the transformation that is part and parcel to their healing.

What I believe and teach is that it is safest to be connected to yourself, because from there you can go anywhere. Also, you need to be first connected to yourself to be able to connect with others. Those are great tag lines, and I use them as such, but they are really what I believe and teach my patients. Those tag lines change lives. They provoke patients into their healing journeys, something they choose for themselves, and then I guide them on their way. Just like the stack of stones by a trail called a *cairn*, the guidance is there to help the patient stay on their path.

So, is there any convention to my practice? Yes. I use electronic medical records. I take a history, vitals, complete an exam, and render a diagnosis and treatment plan. However, that is done in a unique way, with genomics, deep listening and history taking, functional testing, and the treatment of traumatic events that are a component of the patient's life—and frequently the key to helping them heal.

So how does that look? Well, let's dive in and find out.

To Begin a Session of Self Compassion and Connection

Identify what, where, and who you want to explore.

- Was it an incident?
- Was it known?
- Was it unknown?
- Give it a location.
- If a diagnosis is known and felt, use that.

- Score it on a scale of 1-10.

Those questions establish the intention for deeper work and allow permission to access the wisdom of the body. When a session, a meditation, a shamanic journey is started, always start with an intention. That sets the sacred space. It provides guidance to the conscious and unconscious parts of you as well as to your guides, helpers, and spirit source (God, Love, Universe) as to what you are up to. You are establishing the boundaries, and you are in complete control, because you are choosing to enter into the process. No harm can come your way. You are protected.

You may want to journal to begin this session. Jot things down—bullet points, not a diatribe. Not an essay. Just bullet points, so you can return to your thoughts after your session.

When I did this kind of work with my gestalt therapist, I often sent them a summary before my session. That allowed both of us to set the intentions for the session, and it also eliminated a lot of "catching up" since the last session. By checking in with the therapist in this way, they always felt that I got "all my money's worth" in each session from such preparation. I wasn't looking for that; I was intent on healing and moving through the process. That for sure, was accomplished.

The process of my work comes from not only the work I've developed from seeing patients, but also from receiving excellent therapy as I worked through some very difficult situations I experienced in my life. You might be able to say that comes from a "physician, heal thyself" approach. To which my response would be, "Well, if it works for me, it will work for you, so let's go and get 'er done."

Here is how we "get 'er done." See below for the way forward by going inward as an approach to self-healing.

Complete the Self Compassion and Connection (SCAc) Phrases

This establishes the biofield.

Technique: Hold your heart and solar plexus as a gesture of self-connection while going through the SCAC statement:

- "Even though I feel [emotion, or name the situation],
  - I deeply and completely love, trust, and accept myself.
  - I choose to connect or re-connect with myself.

Complete the above cycle three times. With each cycle breathe in and out with this pattern:

- Cycle 1: Breathe in for three seconds and then breathe out for six seconds. One cycle of breathing.
  - Cycle 2: Breathe in for three seconds and then breathe out for six seconds. <u>Repeat two breaths in this cycle because it is cycle two.</u>
  - Cycle 3: Breathe in for three seconds, then breathe out for six seconds. Repeat three breaths total in this cycle because it is cycle three.

Using a Felt Sense for Self-Healing

The SELF acronym provides a gentle, actionable framework:

1. *Sense* the body's subtle messages.

2. *Explore* the emotions tied to these sensations.
3. *Listen* to those insights with compassion and love yourself through them.
4. *Free* the flow of energy and allow healing to unfold.

This approach beautifully aligns with the principles of felt-sense work, trauma-informed care, and integrative healing, offering a holistic path to self-discovery and wellness for patients.

Here are some additional tips about the SELF framework:

S—Sense the Body

- Tune in to the physical sensations within your body. Engage with the *felt sense*, that subtle, nonverbal bodily awareness that holds the key to deeper emotions or unresolved issues.
- Techniques:
  - Take a moment to pause, close your eyes, and scan your body for tension or sensations.
  - Ask yourself, *What am I feeling in my body, and where do I feel it?*
- Importance:
  - This step honors the wisdom of your body and provides the gateway to subconscious processing.

E—Explore Emotions

- Once you've connected with the bodily sensation, explore the emotions or memories tied to it.

Approach this step with curiosity and compassion.

- Techniques:
  - Use open-ended questions, like: *What is this sensation trying to tell me?* or *What does this need?*
  - Reframe anxiety or discomfort as a messenger, not an enemy.
- Importance:
  - By naming and understanding emotions, you create space for healing and insight.

L—Listen and Love

- Deeply listen to what emerges, without judgment, and respond with self-compassion. Embrace the idea that healing begins with reconnecting to yourself.
- Importance:
  - Listening , accepting, and loving yourself creates the safety needed for healing. It also reinforces the connection between mind, body, and spirit.

F—Free the Flow

- Release the stored energy or emotion that was identified. This can involve physical, emotional, or energetic shifts.
- Techniques:
  - Engage in somatic release.
  - Use energetic practices or biofield alignment with the SCAC technique.

  - Reevaluate the SUD (Subjective Unit of Distress) to measure progress. On a scale from one to ten, how is that emotion, sensation, event landing with you now? The goal is to move the needle from a high number, which is usually greater than a 7, to a low number which is 1 or 0. Achieving that indicates a resolution of this symptom, issue, or event, along with a re-connection back to your self. The dissociation was decreased or eliminated.
- Importance:
  - By freeing blocked energy, you restore the body's innate ability to self-regulate and heal. No more shut-down survival mode (autonomic fight, flight, freeze, or fawn). You are in the neuro-regulated zone of "normal" and balanced, feeling and being more connected to yourself as well as aware and able to use tools of resiliency.

Decades ago, the self-help movement emerged. That was a significant step forward. But we face a different set of issues now, as there is so much help, not so much healing. There are a lot of influencers, but not a lot of real experts; lots of ideas, but not a lot of healing; lots of misinformation, and not as much information rooted in integrity regarding its roots, origins, or outcomes. It is kinda like a medical free-for-all, without the benefit of what free-medical-for-all actually could mean. With the rise of social media, there is a lot of misinformation, malinformation, and disinformation. The key is finding and following trusted sources for your true information.

Why should we seek self-healing versus self-help? Don't

we need all of the help we can get? Yes, but let's go beyond help, let's go out there (which is in there—in you) and receive the self-healing.

The table below offers a clear, side-by-side comparison to highlight the fundamental differences between the two approaches.

Aspect	Self-Healing	Self-Help
Focus	Internal, body-centered, and process-driven	Primarily external, often advice- or strategy-based
Goal	Facilitates the body's innate ability to regulate, restore, and rebalance itself	Offers tips or techniques to manage challenges or achieve goals
Approach	Works from the inside out, addressing core issues like trauma, unresolved emotions, and energetic imbalances	Addresses symptoms or surface-level concerns, rather than root causes
Mind-Body Connection	Prioritizes integration of the mind, body, and spirit	Often focuses more on mental strategies, less on embodied awareness
Empowerment	Encourages trust in our own capacity to heal, rather than relying solely on external tools or advice	Can sometimes create dependency on external resources or "fixes"

Not Influenced by Influencers

I don't believe in "the new menopause" or "parts of our selves talking to other parts of ourselves" or "pushing on this spot will stimulate the vagal response and trauma melts away." Those things are just not true. They fall in the category of misinformation or malinformation. I believe in the body's inherent wisdom, which is ancient. I believe in the body's inherent capacity to heal, which is beyond ancient—it's eternal. And I believe we are all individually responsible for our choices and intentions of how we live our lives. That is all-encompassing.

When we experience a traumatic event, our body registers the trauma in the tissues, in the conscious and subconscious, in soul and spirit as well. We are way too complex to have a simple push of a button to make it all go away.

What is interesting is that the system of care that I have created stands on the shoulders of so many who have come and gone before me. It is a vortex of information, intention, and healing wisdom that I draw from. At times, I thought I was being original, but really what I was being was authentic. I was drawing from many things I have learned and researched and used when working with patients. They taught me things by me practicing on them. (Yes, it is the *practice* of medicine, after all.) What happened was that complex issues and techniques seemed to condense, coalesce, and, in a quantum sense, collapse into a simpler way forward. What was complex became simplified. Not easy, and not simple, but simplified. Experiencing that was amazing, and patients began to have some pretty significant healings going forward.

Months-long, years-long, decades-long illnesses, distresses, and diseases began to heal and stay healed. Patients were able to discontinue medications, therapies, and supplements in favor of simply being well again. I too experienced that as a patient myself. I will remind you again of the adage "physician, heal thyself." We may want to expand that one to "physician, experiment on thyself."

As a physician, this is how I now practice. I always believed this way, but I did not always practice this way. What constrained me in the past was the medical system. Working within the medical system wreaked havoc on my intuition and felt sense of who I was as a healer. I would often get called out by administrators for being "different," not one who went with the flow. At times, I was even called disruptive. What is true is that I was different. However, I was not disruptive (to the truth), nor was I going against the flow (of the patient's healing). I was disruptive to the health care system, as the system is not driven by patient care but rather by profit, insurance companies, and pre-established ways of treating one as many. So, yes, guilty on all accounts. Now I am simply outside of the system, working with patients in my own private practice.

It is important in our evolution as humans to know that, as regards our current medical system, what we have is not sustainable. It is obsolete. It is bloated. It is focused on corporate profit and not on the patient. It is reductionistic and not holistic—a pill for an ill and a dismissal of what can't or doesn't fall in line with insurance guidelines and pre-approved or prior-authorized choices. Or, worse, you get all of that *and* you are told that your illness is all in your head, or there must be "something wrong with you!" *Ugh.*

Whoa there, Dr. Louder, not everything in medicine is like that. There are some good doctors and clinics and hospitals and approaches to care. Yes, that is true. There are isolated aberrations to what I am saying. But its roots and core are now coming from corporate medicine, profit-sharing, and insurance guidelines, not personalized medicine. The pendulum has gone too far to one side, and it needs to swing back. Ha. As it does so, it may hit a few administrators and insurance companies in their backsides as it is swinging by.

What I know to be true is that working one-on-one with patients and taking this care model to many others by way of online learning and education, we might just push that pendulum the other direction more quickly. Not really wanting any violence, but I would want to see the current health system restructured into a fully paid-for, patient-centered, and patient- and physician-empowered style of care.

I am concerned that perhaps the only way forward for the medical system may also mean the way inward. There would be an implosion and crumbling of our medical care system, with a birthing of something new. I am not saying this as if I am coming from either political party. Rather, I am coming from the physician/patient view of this, as well as being an advocate for common humanity.

My Soul's Lesson

I was born a catalyst, positive disruptor, and visionary. When I show up, things change, just by me being there. Nothing doing but simply being. This happens across the board in my life, not only in medicine. At all levels, my anatomy is designed to bring healing, to myself and to others.

My soul's work is to see others heal as I have healed. The healing lessons shaped my life and are intimately related. They provided the structure (anatomy) for finding a felt sense, which is the function of awareness, presence, and life, and that is the purpose and experience of my soul (physiology or function).

The fact that I am in medicine as a career and life calling leads me to a full intention to be a part of changing our medical system—one patient, one encounter, one diagnosis at a time. Then moving out from there to groups, communities, and cultures. All the while standing in my full integrity and presence of being.

Employing the doctor/patient relationship, which is built upon a self-healing model of care from a holistic, integrative perspective, is the way forward. It is what I felt as a youngster when I had a felt sense that there was some purpose for my life. It is what I felt as I stood up against the elders to claim my right to become a physician. It is what I had a deep felt sense about when things got tough and I wanted out. I am glad that I did not leave or die, but rather chose to embrace the calling that was always there for me, choosing to live with a felt sense of what I know to do, where I am meant to be, and who I am—a physician and a healer.

www.ingramcontent.com/pod-product-compliance
Lightning Source LLC
LaVergne TN
LVHW022213200926
848481LV00006B/1952